"A very compelling memoir by a wise, curious, insightful physician. He candidly shares his life's story and describes many very touching and, at times, incredibly humorous events. This should be required reading for all medical students and those involved in the field of health care."

—*Edward J. O'Connell, MD*
Emeritus Professor of Pediatrics, Allergy/Immunology, Mayo Clinic College of Medicine
Emeritus Editor in Chief of Annals of Allergy, Asthma and Immunology

"On one level, *Office Upstairs* demonstrates the value of personal story as a vehicle for understanding history, especially as it relates to the practice of medicine, the Jewish experience and the South. On another, it shows the kindness, good humor and ethical values of an eminent physician, a 'mensch' with extraordinary judgment and deep humility."

—*Martin Perlmutter, PhD*
Professor of Philosophy
Director, Yaschik/Arnold Jewish Studies Program, College of Charleston

"Come along for an entertaining and heartwarming ride as seen through the eyes of Charleston's pioneering allergist."

—*Edward M. Gilbreth, MD*
Charleston physician, author and contributor to The Post and Courier

Office Upstairs

A Doctor's Journey

Charles H. Banov, MD

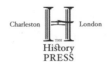

Charleston · London
THE
History
PRESS

Published by The History Press
Charleston, SC 29403
www.historypress.net

Cover design by Marshall Hudson.

Hardcover edition first published 2007.
Paperback edition published in 2008.

Manufactured in the United Kingdom

ISBN 978.1.59629.504.9

Library of Congress CIP data applied for.

Contents

*To my wife, Nancy, who encouraged me to write this story,
and to my patients, who helped me live it.*

Preface

Preface

E very attempt was made in this memoir to ensure accuracy. Since many of the people mentioned are deceased and some of the incidents occurred more than fifty years ago, my personal records, diary, interviews, newspaper clippings, scrapbooks and public records were utilized extensively. When appropriate, fictitious names were given to some of the characters in the stories, but the incidents described were recorded as remembered and documented.

Acknowledgements

I appreciate the help given me in preparation of this book by my children, Drs. Mark and Michael Banov and Lori Banov Kaufmann, as well as my son-in-law Yadin Kaufmann and daughter-in-law Lisa Banov. The suggestions of my sisters, Caren Masem and Linda Stern, and my brother-in-law, Dr. Paul Masem, were helpful. I thank Oprah Winfrey for her suggestion that I write a book in the first place. I am grateful for the advice given me by my classmate Dr. Walter Bonner, who is also an author; my colleague Dr. Curtis Worthington Jr., director of the Waring Historical Library; historian Robert Rosen; author Jack Bass; journalist Sandy Katz; physician/writer Dr. Edward M. Gilbreth; as well as editors Professor Carol Anne Davis and Lynne McNeil and my major editors, Anne Kostick and Stephen Hoffius.

However, a special thank you goes to my daughter Pamela, who because of her mental disability could not read the manuscript and will never be able to do so. But I thank her for teaching us that there is a meaningful life to be lived and enjoyed by every human being. While writing the book I derived my greatest encouragement and strength from the only contribution she could make: the gift of a smile!

Introduction
A Memorable Walk

In April 1993, I was asked to participate in a postgraduate course at the lovely Camelback resort in Scottsdale, Arizona. On the first evening, the recreation staff offered a nature walk into the desert areas near the resort as a before-dinner exercise. A small group of walkers assembled. All of them seemed like the usual type of guest at an elegant resort, except for one woman. She was not wearing designer clothes; she had a kerchief on her head, a white T-shirt and blue exercise tights. My wife Nancy recalls those details; all I remember is that she had very large sunglasses. She was walking by herself, and I had the feeling that the other guests were avoiding her.

I felt some empathy for her, so I decided to walk along with her and try to make her feel comfortable. She proved to be a charming conversationalist. I pointed out all the celebrity homes I knew of in the area, and she appeared interested.

She asked about my home in Charleston. She said she had visited our city recently and enjoyed it very much. We talked about my work as a physician in the South. When I told her some of my stories, she suggested that I write a book about my experiences. I had not really considered writing a book, but I thought, *If this lady finds my stories interesting, maybe I should do it.* I thought it was fortunate that I had chosen to keep her company. I filed "write a book" in my mental list of things to do.

My wife walked with another group. When we returned to the resort, I bid farewell to my companion and rejoined Nancy and our friends. I apologized for having spent the entire walk with this lady. I explained that she was by herself, and I'd felt sorry for her.

"Do you know whom you were walking with?" Nancy asked me.

"No," I replied.

She gave me a look of disbelief. "That was Oprah Winfrey!"

After dinner that night, Ms. Winfrey appeared for her lecture elegantly dressed, poised, charming and perfectly recognizable.

So I can honestly lay the responsibility for this book's existence on Oprah's suggestion that I write down my stories. Blame her.

Chapter 1

The Early Years
Growing Up in the South

A cartoonist once depicted an announcement from proud Jewish parents proclaiming the birth of their child. The card proclaimed the name of the baby "Dr. _____." Perhaps I was not born a doctor, as the cartoon implied, but my curious adventures in medicine certainly began that early.

I was delivered by a veterinarian. I doubt that this was what my mother intended when she went to the hospital to give birth to me, but I was a breech baby, the family doctor was having a hard time and the specialist on duty, who happened to be in the building, also happened to be a veterinarian. In spite of the implications of entering the world ass-backward at the hands of a horse doctor, I've always felt lucky: after all, it might've been a dentist.

This was in Charleston, South Carolina, in 1930. Charleston is one of the most interesting and beautiful cities in America. It has been the home of the largest Jewish community of colonial times, with roots going back to the 1690s; an early commercial center with a very cosmopolitan, cultured atmosphere; an important location in the War Between the States, from the firing on Fort Sumter that launched the war to the city's capture by Union forces four years later. Charleston has survived economic depressions and economic revivals, a major earthquake in 1886 and several powerful hurricanes.

My father, Milton Banov, was born here, as was his mother. They were part of the tightly knit Jewish community, which by the 1930s had been greatly enlarged by recent immigrants from Eastern Europe, including my grandfathers. In Jewish Charleston, to have a grandmother who was born here was rare. We went back quite far. My father was very proud of the family's history here and he was very proud of being American. I have inherited his love of Charleston's history as well as his frustrated aspirations to be its official tour guide.

There was always one doctor in the Jewish community. He was the one who performed circumcisions, deliveries and so forth. But for less dire or less expensive medical help, the immigrants went to my grandfather, Sam Banov.

Sam Banov was a sort of quasi-doctor; he had no medical training, but he did have a big medical book. People came to his clothing store with their complaints. He consulted the book and then gave them various medicines.

One time, somebody came in with what turned out to be an inflamed appendix. My grandfather prescribed a laxative and the appendix ruptured. Grandfather was so distraught that the surgeon (the aforementioned Jewish doctor) brought my grandfather into the operating room to let him see that the fellow was all right. But Grandfather was very upset about having missed the diagnosis; that may have been when he stopped practicing medicine and relegated the big medical book to the attic.

As a teenager, I discovered the book and spent hours up there, absorbed in reading it. The big book may have led to my interest in homegrown research experiments. I remember in high school I hid various types of weeds under my father's pillow and then made a scientific record of his sneezing the next morning.

Even before that time, doctors and medicine held my interest. My childhood stories included Dr. Doolittle in books, Dr. Kildare in the movies and Dr. Christian in the early 1940s radio show. When I was seven years old, I found an injured turtle in the park. Since these were the pre-EMS years, I transported the animal in the luxurious facility of my back pocket. I took the turtle down to my office in the basement and performed major, and probably innovative, surgical procedures, which saved the turtle's life—or so I thought. My complex medical therapy consisted of applying, with just the right touch, a mixture of Mercurochrome and iodine. The frightened turtle finally projected his head from the shell, and I believed that I was responsible for a medical miracle. But, as I was to learn on many occasions in the future, patients—and turtles—often get well despite their doctors. It was probably not until college, when I took a course in comparative anatomy, that I began to question whether my ministrations to this turtle were as lifesaving as I thought. The turtle never let on.

Charleston back in those days was a comfortable, predictable city, easy to live in. My life was bound by the social conventions and religious obligations of the Jewish community, as well as those of a segregated Southern state.

I spent a lot of time at the library, partly because of the wonderful librarian Janey Smith (known to us as Miss Janey), who looked just like a librarian in the movies, with glasses and her hair in a bun. But even if I might have been a bit of what's now called a nerd, I still had to fight. Fighting was a big part of being a Southern schoolboy in those days. Bullies ruled the schoolyard, and the teachers encouraged these confrontations. When we had fights, we were sent to the gymnasium and the whole school was called to witness it. It happened to me.

Two brothers, notorious bullies, always picked on me when I left school on my bicycle in the afternoon. I put up with this for a few months until one day, when they threw my bike down as usual. I said, "Did you throw my bike down?" and one of the brothers said, "Yeah. What are you going to do about it?" I fought him immediately, and won. The next day I fought the other brother. I had to do this for three or four days, alternating brothers, with the whole school watching. When I got home I tried to hide my hands, which were swollen from fighting. I used liniment on them all weekend because I knew I'd have to come back Monday and fight again. It was hard, but after that they left me alone. Many years later, I heard that one of them grew up to be a prizefighter and the other was convicted of murder. Had I been able to peek into the future, perhaps I wouldn't have taken them on.

My friends were the other Jewish boys in town, who I met in school or at synagogue. I can't say that fighting bullies (or ministering to myself in the aftermath) made me want to become a doctor, but growing up in an atmosphere of high regard for professionals, with medicine as the pinnacle of all professions, certainly had its influence.

As Jews, we always knew we were different. In Charleston, this was even more the case: in spite of our long history there, we were neither part of white Charleston society nor of the equally historical black community. As the other communities pretty much kept to themselves, so did we.

Both my grandfather and my father were storekeepers in the poorer sections of town. A certain level of crime was endemic. There were gangs then, as now, which came in, took things off the shelves and disrupted the business. My grandfather was told he should defend himself. Most Jewish immigrants in those days were gentle people when it came to physical actions; they didn't fight back. But the other merchants said it was the only thing he could do. They gave him a blackjack, which was a club covered with leather and small enough to keep hidden. The next person who came in and bothered him, my grandfather just went at him with the blackjack. He never had another problem with the gangs. I inherited his blackjack. I like to think his spirit came down to me too, and helped me defeat those schoolyard bullies.

I encountered few black people in my younger years. We had a maid, Susie Gathers, who lived on Moultrie Street, four or five houses down from us. She used to babysit me, which meant that she sat on the edge of my bed and stayed there until my parents came home. She used to plan all our meals and do the cooking, and we didn't find out until just a few months before she died that she was illiterate. She had a daughter who was the same age as my younger sister Linda, and the two grew up together as friends. They didn't recognize any difference between themselves until they got into their teens. They went to different, segregated schools. Society began teaching them its lessons, and it became obvious that the world would not offer the same opportunities to both. They stayed friends, but only marginally.

Growing up Jewish may have heightened my sensitivity to other aspects of Charleston without my realizing it. I was probably about fifteen years old, and Rosa Parks's act of defiance of the typical segregation laws of the South was still a decade in the future, when one day I boarded a city bus to go downtown. A few stops later, an elderly black woman climbed, with difficulty, the front steps of the bus and began her walk to the back, the "colored" section, which for her was a considerable distance. I was sitting close to the front; there was an empty seat next to me. As she came toward me, I said, "Come sit by me," and helped her into the vacant third-row seat. My action didn't seem extraordinary to me. My father had instilled a respect for elders that did not recognize racial boundaries or, apparently, legal ones. By offering her a seat at the front of the bus, I helped a little old lady break the law.

About two blocks later, the driver stopped the bus and, with real anger, made me get out. As I trudged home, I was scared to death of what my father's reaction might be. It wasn't that I'd never been in trouble, but somehow this brush with authority felt more serious than anything that had happened before.

I hadn't noticed that one of our neighbors (a retired marine corps colonel, and as redneck as they come) had been on the bus with me and witnessed the entire incident. There was plenty of time during my long walk home for him to call my father and tell him about his smart-ass kid, who the driver had wisely thrown off the bus as a lesson for the future. He thought my father would want to commend the driver.

But he didn't know my father, a true Southern gentleman without a prejudiced bone in his body. As I approached the house my dread increased with every step. It doubled when I spotted my father walking briskly from the backyard with the same stern face he'd had when I was caught a year earlier selling illegal firecrackers. He grabbed me fiercely by the shoulders. I saw tears in his eyes, felt a tremor through his hands and was sure he was angrier with me than he'd ever been in his life. Then I found myself enveloped in a huge bear hug and heard him utter one word, the best a son can hear from a father: "Mensch!"

We never mentioned the incident again.

For those of us who were children in the 1940s and too young for the military, the decade was a period of intense patriotism. Before Pearl Harbor, sailors from the Charleston Naval Base were rarely welcomed to respectable Charleston homes. Families might attend parties with servicemen, but their daughters were not encouraged to date them. All of this changed on December 7, 1941. Suddenly, everyone in uniform was a hero, and our homes were opened to those who had previously been called "nasty, beer-drinking sailors"; now they were son-in-law material.

We followed World War II as if it were a football series. Clearly, we were the good guys, winning exciting battles on land, on sea and in Saturday-afternoon, nine-cent movies. The bad guys were easily identified, not just by their black hats, but also because they were so ugly compared to the white hats such as Clark Gable and James Stewart. For the first two years of the war, I basked in the thrills and comradeship of watching military parades and singing patriotic songs on Charleston streets. Perhaps our token sacrifices of rationed gasoline and allowances of two pairs of new shoes a year helped me think that I was sharing the fight with all of the other kids of the world.

But medicine and war had a way of intersecting in my life more than once. If I believed in omens, I might have spotted some unseen hand (besides my mother's) steering me in the direction of a medical career.

When I was a twelve-year-old camper at a Boy Scout camp near Charleston, a large group of us took advantage of an unusually low tide to wade into the mud of a tidal creek in search of fiddler crabs. Suddenly, the beach around the pluff mud resembled the Normandy invasion. Practically every camper, including me, was lacerated by hidden, very sharp oyster shells. It was a bloody beachhead!

Unknown to my fellow campers and especially my school friends (to whom I did not want to appear to be a sissy), I had attended a special civil defense course with my mother. I had learned about the application of pressure on wounds to stop bleeding and about how to organize a group of casualties into self-help units so that they could assist each other until medical help arrived. Because the Red Cross instructor was reluctant to have a child in his adult course, my mother had to plead to get me admitted. In the end, he was no match for the intensity of my mother's passion to groom me to be a doctor.

Down on the beach, I set to work. With towels, sheets and any other makeshift dressing, I got my fellow campers' bleeding under control. The camp director, who had been in Charleston attending a meeting, returned about then, and although concerned about the mishap, he was also relieved and surprised that the "mess" had been handled by one of his twelve-year-old Scouts. He was probably most worried about drawing criticism for lax supervision.

They say that everyone has his fifteen minutes of fame. As a result of the "action on the beach," as someone called it, I was given special recognition at the annual Boy Scout banquet some months later. Since there was no appropriate medal for a child directing a beach rescue activity, I was awarded a lapel pin meant for medical professionals for outstanding medical services to the Boy Scouts of America.

I loved that pin and was extremely proud of it, especially since it had the caduceus on it. I must have gazed at that pin every hour, right through the night. My mother could relax now—I was hooked on medicine.

About three months later, I received a telephone call from the regional director of the Boy Scouts. It was about that pin. The local branch had made an error; the pin could only be given to a real physician and I would have to return it. Instead, the regional director would give me a more practical gift—a wristwatch with a second hand, something that was still relatively new in the world. I would certainly be the only kid on my block to have a green Boy Scout wristwatch, but I wanted my pin!

I surrendered it to the regional director and received my obviously expensive watch in return. I hoped no one saw the tears in my eyes.

To this day, each morning when I search for my socks in my dresser drawer I come upon a box filled with useless lapel pins, given during a lifetime of personal and professional community service. I'd be happy to throw them all away, and probably will one of these days. No matter what kind of recognition I've received in whatever form, I would have preferred to have that little pin with the symbol of the physician. It was another ten years before I became eligible to wear it, but I was never again given the chance.

When I was about fifteen years old and started to read sections of the newspaper other than the comics, I began to understand that people were getting hurt in this war and perhaps I should be doing more for the war effort than collecting old rubber tires. My adventuresome cousin Norman Arnold and I hatched a plan to stow away on a hospital ship, save lives and help win the war, all without any danger of getting hurt ourselves, of course. Our elaborate plans consumed about one hour on the morning of our caper and included such logistics as the preparation of three corned beef sandwiches apiece.

A few bottles of Coke and a Baby Ruth candy bar were added to carry us through the transatlantic crossing to the battlefields. Missing from our strategic planning was the idea of notifying our parents. That was unimportant; they'd read all about it in the papers. If we had to miss school, too bad! We were vague in our own minds about what services we would perform on the ship. My medical skills were still limited to reading Grandpa Banov's book and practicing on that turtle. And since neither of us would consent to helping our families around the house, we would be no good at swabbing decks.

Hospital ships are impressive-looking vessels—painted white, with massive red crosses on the decks. We had visited the Charleston Naval Shipyard many times and knew exactly where to locate the hospital ships that were in for repair. Admittance to the shipyard was easy—all one had to do was not look German or Japanese. Looking Japanese wasn't a problem. We were certain we'd never be taken for German spies because we knew that all Germans looked like Adolph Hitler and had his funny haircut. So, with perfect confidence, we simply walked up the gangplank and onto the ship. Two armed guards thought it was nice that we were delivering sandwiches to our uncle. We were so convincing that they never bothered to ask his name.

We decided to hide out in a large, extremely clean section of a room that did, upon reflection, seem a bit isolated. In fact, it was the poison gas decontamination unit. Any crewmember coming upon us there would not doubt for a minute that we were out of bounds, and that's what happened not long after we arrived.

The captain was on leave, so we were taken to the executive officer. Fortunately for us, the exec had children of his own—six, in fact—none with any imagination. So he gave us a guided tour with all the flourishes, a tour usually reserved for visiting navy or political brass. The day finished with an invitation to the mess hall for dinner.

Everyone was so friendly that I was beginning to think about the next military facility we might unofficially visit. Then our host showed us one last room, which surprised me because I didn't know it existed on a hospital ship. It was the brig. The exec told us flatly that this would be our fate should we ever again set foot on any other ship in wartime without permission.

We didn't.

C:>

I confess I hadn't always wanted to become a doctor. What I really wanted to be when I grew up was a policeman or a detective. The movies and radio shows of the '40s helped convince me. In those stories, policemen and detectives solved puzzles, pursued the truth and aided in the triumph of Good over Evil. But as a career path, law enforcement wasn't my family's first choice for me. In the years during and after World War II, Jewish families seemed to share a particular overriding aspiration for their sons—a profession that allowed them to be self-employed and not subject to the whims of an employer who might have anti-Semitic feelings. This meant medicine or law. My family was no different. It wasn't until I had been a specialist for some years that I realized how much the field of allergy is like the detective business—the only difference, perhaps, is that the bad guys don't shoot back.

I pursued my medical degree with the intensity of Dick Tracy hot on a criminal's trail. At Emory University in Atlanta, I majored in Getting into Medical School, and I was not alone in that department.

The fraternities supported each other across college lines too. Although some of our joint activities were pure *Animal House*, we were not unaware of the serious political and social issues of the day. In fact, we felt them keenly. Civil rights, politics and the future of our country were topics of heated debate.

Those were the days of the Talmadge era: Governor Eugene Talmadge, with his trademark red suspenders, waving a shotgun and followed in office by his son, Herman Talmadge. Both men personified the rabid Southern segregationist. Those years saw the beginning of the battle between the federal government's push to legislate and enforce fair employment practices, desegregation and civil rights, and the South's fierce, often violent resistance. The battle continued for more than two decades.

In 1948, Henry Wallace, who had been vice president in the Roosevelt administration, ran for president on the Progressive Party ticket. He advocated an end to segregation, as well as voting rights for blacks. He came to Atlanta, amid many threats, to speak at a black church. We Emory students got in touch with some black students at Morehouse College. They helped us sneak past the angry picketers (who would likely have tarred and feathered any whites they caught entering the church) in order to hear Wallace speak.

For the black students, the threat of violence was nothing to ignore: the state of Georgia, along with Mississippi, led the nation in lynchings. Those were the days of the Ku Klux Klan and cross burnings. We wanted to help fight back, and actually attended a few cross burnings, bringing along our fraternity brothers, the big football players from the Georgia Tech chapter. Each of our boys stood next to a Klansman, looming over him as the evening progressed. It was meant as counter-intimidation, and it worked.

Most of the time, we studied and schemed. Those of us majoring in Med School (Getting In) were pathologically concerned about our grade point averages. What we really needed was an easy course (nonscientific, naturally) to boost that magic number. We decided to register for a Bible study class—how difficult could it be?

But there was a problem. While the average Christian student had enough familiarity with the Bible to guarantee an A with little effort, we Jewish pre-meds had stopped our religious education at our bar mitzvah, or at least at the end of the Old Testament.

To create equality in grading, we resorted to the age-old custom of buttering up the teacher. Mr. Julius Newman was a withdrawn, insecure missionary's son who had spent twenty-five of his thirty years in the socially void confines of various Asian church schools. We invited him to dinner at our fraternity house, where he was introduced to the forbidden temptations of beer and pornography (the marijuana of the 1950s). Eventually he confided that not only was he a virgin, but he had never had a single date with a girl and didn't even know how to begin a conversation on a nonreligious subject.

What an opportunity for us!

Mr. Newman was too honorable to repay our attention and friendship with an undeserved high grade, but he did agree to a trade: he would coach us, in a formal, remedial way, on what we needed to know to excel in the course. In return, we would teach him how to approach the innocent female instructor in his department. I can still see the blackboard in the fraternity house: on one side was a list of the apostles, on the other side our advice: "Touch her hand gently in the movie, but don't put your arm around her until you get her in the car."

Everyone in our fraternity who took the class made an honest A, and Mr. Newman invited the entire fraternity to his wedding. His wife never knew that he came to the fraternity house after each date for a critique of the evening. Our coaching ended with the wedding, but apparently we were the best of mentors: the couple went on to have four beautiful children, and he did that all on his own.

The Early Years: Growing Up in the South

In my last year at Emory, I shared an apartment off-campus with a fellow pre-med student. Our landladies were two elderly sisters with tremendous maternal instincts, who would always bring us glasses of warm milk and sandwiches at night to encourage us as we studied.

My roommate and I were cramming for a final exam in comparative anatomy, one of those must-ace courses for any aspiring medical student. A main teaching tool for that course was an embalmed cat, well marked with latex strips labeling specific organs and blood vessels. Students were required to memorize its internal details. I decided to bring my cat back to my room so I could study all night. I was happy to see my milk and sandwich waiting for me on my desk.

Sitting at my desk at the far end of our room, my back was to the hallway door. That night the sweet little ladies came in to say goodnight. When they opened the door, all they could see was my back as I bent over my desk, with a cat head on the left, the cat's legs sticking out on the right and the sound of my jaws working as I vigorously chewed my corned beef sandwich while using a probe to review the various parts of the cat's anatomy.

The sweet little ladies survived the shock and claimed never to have believed for a second that I was eating a cat, but the next year they began renting the room exclusively to theology students. I got an A on the final.

Atlanta is 340 miles from Charleston, but it might have been across the ocean in the view of a callow teenager. In Atlanta I grew up quickly. Still, there was a lot to learn about the way the world worked.

I was taking a political science course and was casting around for a term paper topic. It's no surprise that at that point my academic interest intersected my other burning interest—dancing to the tune played by my raging hormones.

And, although I was then in college, I must have still wanted to be a policeman. When the course required me to interview someone in government, I chose the police department.

Atlanta was not unusual among big cities in having a well-established sex industry that catered to all ages and interests. (As I was to discover, my own hometown had a fine tradition in this regard.) Fraternity boys were a major source of revenue in certain Atlanta brothels that specialized in relieving these kids of their virginity.

I went to the police department and, in the course of the interview, informed the inspector that prostitution existed in his city. He said he knew it.

"But there are numerous establishments operating in full view of the authorities, who must be bribed to look the other way. They're corrupting the morals of minors," I told them.

"Really?" replied the inspector, looking astonished.

I offered my services as an undercover detective. He accepted. For the next few weeks, I "investigated" the brothels of Atlanta, on behalf (I thought) of Emory University and the Atlanta Police Department. Two or three times I reported my findings to a grateful (I thought) police department. When my work became known to the world at large, I would be famous (I thought).

Then the dean called me into his office. The police department had had enough of me, apparently, and the inspector told the dean to get this kid out of their hair. The dean explained the real facts of life to me: you don't expose corruption in Atlanta.

I got an A on the term paper, although to my surprise it didn't make me famous. And they had a big laugh in the police department.

For me, college was a trade school. I spent my four years training to be a medical school applicant, instead of acquiring a true liberal arts education, or learning to think about the world. In college, I learned to do surgery on a grasshopper, but I haven't been called upon to do that in the more than fifty years since. Nor did the experience enlarge my understanding of the world or help make me a good person. That was my loss. Pre-med students are entitled to a wonderful, well-rounded education in all disciplines, especially the humanities. In the end, it will make them better doctors.

In 1951, my last year at Emory, the finish line was in sight. It wasn't hard to handicap the medical school horse race: few girls were ever accepted, blacks never were and at the Medical College of South Carolina, there was an unwritten but obvious rule that limited the number of Jewish applicants accepted. For the past one hundred years there were usually two, but occasionally up to four, Jews accepted in any class. Every bright, Jewish, pre-med student in the state competed for those few places. This is quite different from the present time, as the school has a Jewish president and a Jewish dean of graduate studies. Although practically everybody I knew at Emory was pre-med, they would apply to different medical schools. I knew I was really competing only against the other South Carolina Jewish students.

As a backup, I had applied to the Federal Bureau of Investigation for a position as a fingerprint technician. This would provide some scientific training and satisfy my desire to be a policeman/detective/undercover agent.

It was the height of the Korean conflict and the military draft was operating full steam. If I made it into medical school, I'd be the hero of the day. If I didn't make it, I'd be drafted. In fact, I'd already been drafted, but not yet called.

My medical school application had been submitted months before—it was probably the first one that the school received—but by May I still had not received a response. On a depressing Friday afternoon, after visiting my mailbox for another disappointing non-response, I received a telephone call from FBI headquarters requesting that I come down the next morning for a formal interview. With the fear of a Communist behind every bush, I assumed that the FBI screening process was very thorough. This seemed a strange way to schedule an interview—giving me only half a day to prepare and without sending a formal letter of request. Naturally, I suspected another Georgia Tech fraternity prank, but decided it must be the real thing.

The next morning I arrived at 8:30 a.m., expecting to see the very dramatic, efficient and massive FBI office. After all, Atlanta was the district headquarters for the bureau. Instead, I was ushered into a very small, compact room with two desks and two typewriters, complete with two unsmiling typists who were banging away at their machines. At first they hardly acknowledged me, but as time passed it became harder to ignore me. We were together all morning as I waited for my official interviewer. The two typists were as friendly as they could be under the awkward circumstances. They offered me a soft drink and inquired politely about my fraternity house, friends and schoolwork. They apologized profusely for the special agent, who never appeared.

Finally, after almost four hours of sitting in the cramped quarters and being asked a number of embarrassing questions, including some about my sex life, I was led into the district director's office for my interview. When I opened the door, I saw dozens of desks, file cabinets and office machines clattering; about what I would expect for a major district FBI headquarters.

After I introduced myself, the director said, "Well, thanks very much for coming. You will hear from us."

"But, sir," I explained, "I'm supposed to have my interview."

"Oh, you already had your interview," he replied. "Four hours of it, by our two agents." Two very well-trained agents, that is, posing as typists. Doubtless, they conducted one of the most candid interviews one could possibly have, and I fell for the entire scheme.

I must not have revealed anything too alarming though, as I was offered a position a few weeks later. But by then, my medical school acceptance had at last arrived, and my dream was realized. I would become a doctor.

Chapter 2

Medical School and Beyond

A t last I was a medical student, on my way to becoming a real doctor. I was back in my hometown, living in my childhood home and the world was about to open up for me. I'd been waiting for this all my life.

During our first orientation session, I met a student who would become one of my best medical school friends. Julian Atkinson was from the upper part of the state and a graduate of The Citadel Military College, but he was quite the opposite of the square-shouldered, self-confident, rigid, military school–type so many of us imagine. He was a country boy, a hunting-and-fishing Baptist (without the Bible quoting) who had probably never been farther than twelve miles from home. He was a wonderful member of our four-man anatomy team, and he was the only person in the class more nervous than I, or more compulsive, although he would never admit it.

As medical students, Julian and I shared a special part-time job. On Saturday mornings, we were paid ten dollars to drive more than five hours to Columbia, the state capital, in the Medical College truck and bring back the cadavers of unclaimed bodies from the state mental hospital. In those days, there was no interstate highway, and we had to pick up some ice to keep the cadavers cool. I'll always remember the look on the faces of the ice workers when we drove our truck in, opened the box and said, "Please give us a load of ice before we go fishing."

During one Saturday morning cadaver run, we stopped in the town of Holly Hill so Julian could visit the restroom and buy a pack of cigarettes. As I waited in the truck, I heard a tap on the door. It was a hitchhiker we had passed about a mile back. He asked if he could have a ride to Charleston. I explained that we were medical students taking some cadavers to the school, so there was really no place for him to sit. The hitchhiker said that was fine with him; he himself was a pre-med student. He would be happy to ride in the back.

The young man climbed in the back of the truck. When Julian returned I either forgot to tell him that we had a hitchhiker or, more likely, couldn't resist the opportunity of giving my friend the fright of his life. We'd gone a few miles down the highway when Julian opened his pack of cigarettes. Our passenger, who could see us in the front seat through a glass window, decided he'd like a smoke too. He tapped on the window, and Julian swallowed his cigarette. To this day, I believe I saw cigarette smoke coming out his nostrils.

Much of the time we medical students affected an irreverent, jokey attitude toward the part of our education that had to do with dead human bodies. Of course, our so-called humor was our way of deflecting our unease at dealing with the human body.

We named our cadaver Ernest (because we were working "in dead earnest"). Not everyone appreciated our sense of humor. The three female students in our class were not amused at all when, the first night after receiving our cadaver, while they were washing the body, we childishly made disrespectful comments about their having been issued a male specimen. Although cadaver naming may still go on, our other pranks would now be considered unacceptable by students. Fortunately, on my third day of medical school, I received one of the most dramatic lessons in all my four years.

The anatomy laboratory housed multiple sets of skeletons and partial skeletons. These teaching materials were fragile, and at the beginning of each school year the broken parts were collected and incinerated. We students saw an opportunity for a souvenir—portions of the skull made marvelous ashtrays.

Our anatomy professor had spotted the loot protruding from our briefcases and back pockets as we left the lab. The next day, when we were all assembled for the morning lecture, the professor brought out the box that held the bones. He was so upset that his fiery red face suggested an impending stroke and his usually disciplined posture assumed the position of a coiled rattlesnake about to strike.

"These bones were once part of a human being," he said. "Perhaps they once supported a mother worried about her children because she was, no doubt, a pauper. When she died, her body came to us because her family could not afford her mortuary expenses. Or the bones may have belonged to a patient who suffered from a painful illness that ultimately killed him. Had he lived longer, medical science might have found a way to save him."

Our professor firmly informed us that if we could not, at this early stage in our career, respect a dead human body, we would never be able to understand and appreciate a live one.

"Imagine whatever you like about the person your cadaver may once have been, the pleasures and disappointments that were experienced by the person it once was. But if you cannot treat the dead with consideration for who they were in life, please leave the classroom immediately. There is no place in medicine for you."

That was all it took. We never spoke of it again, but none of us ever forgot it.

A skeleton was one kind of medical school teaching model. When I was a student, we had another kind as well. We had Miss Fanny Warshavsky.

Today, medical education has sophisticated teaching devices at its disposal. In addition to computers, there are elegantly constructed mechanical mannequins that can be programmed to simulate patients with various diseases. We had none of these devices, but we did have live patients, such as Miss Fanny, eager to demonstrate their symptoms. They were rewarded, if not with a medical cure, then by having a permanent home and plenty of sympathetic students to listen to their problems and take an interest in them.

The thought of a patient with a chronic disease living in a hospital and receiving expensive care for years is almost unimaginable today, but Miss Fanny was such a patient. She had developed severe and crippling rheumatoid arthritis, and had come to live quite comfortably in the hospital. She could neither walk nor feed herself, but she helped teach thousands of students about this most painfully deforming disease, as well as about courage and strength.

Miss Fanny patiently demonstrated the ravages of her disease to students, interns and residents in language that each could understand, depending on the stage of his training. Many a candidate for a specialization in internal medicine was examined at her bedside, and woe unto the inconsiderate student who unceremoniously threw off her bedcovers, failed to introduce himself or showed the lack of respect for a charity hospital patient that was pervasive among many medical students at certain stages of their careers. She had no compunction about feeding incorrect answers to a student she did not like, or, for one she did approve of, fully preparing him with the questions she knew would be asked. She was both a teaching machine and a human set of crib notes. All of her students left school with special knowledge about rheumatoid arthritis. More importantly, they never forgot the person with the disease. There were a few other resident teachers in our wards, although no one as memorable as Miss Fanny.

My mother had introduced me to Miss Fanny when I was ten years old, and I began visiting her as part of my family's plan to steer me to a career in medicine. No one was prouder than she when I first came into her ward wearing my medical student's white coat. I know she was proud because when we received our white coats, my family and I stood in front of the mirror for a full five minutes; Miss Fanny had me stand there for fifteen minutes. I never told anyone, but actually I had stood alone in front of the mirror admiring myself for twice that time. In the history of medicine, no stethoscope was fitted in so many positions in two pockets of a medical jacket and admired in such detail. I truly believe it was Miss Fanny's connections with the angels of heaven that secured my acceptance to medical school.

My memory of medical school consists mostly of people rather than events. Not only people, but pictures of people framed in sequence, as in a comic strip. When I remember them, it's as if I were reading their stories in the little balloons above the pictures.

For example, Dr. Andrews was a researcher and part-time instructor in anatomy. He was an "interesting" person, which euphemistically means we found him a little strange. He didn't socialize very much with humans—in fact his hobby, social life and research were devoted entirely to the psychology and well-being of apes.

Dr. Andrews had a federal grant to study a group of chimps, which were allowed to share his life and daily activities. He shunned intimate contact with humans, so there was no danger of his acquiring a wife to interfere with this research. It was not unusual for Dr. Andrews to take his subjects to drive-in movies or fast-food establishments, so most of the city was aware of this unusual research project at the Medical College.

Since my family occasionally invited my friends for dinner, I brought Dr. Andrews and two of his better-behaved chimps home for a kosher Friday night dinner. I don't recall most of the details of the evening, except that my mother insisted that the chimps wear yarmulkes to appease my grandmother, who was very much the traditionalist.

Much of what I learned during medical school was not on the formal curriculum, such as a very dramatic lesson I received on the power of belief. During my relatively innocent young life, I had never experienced drugs. I had barely even heard of marijuana until our second course of pharmacology. There, on the shelf of our laboratory, sat a massive, translucent bowl labeled "Cannabis. Do Not Disturb."

I was curious as to what it would be like to smoke some of this material, and not just from a scientific standpoint. What would this do to enhance my weekend enjoyment, and what fun would I have smoking something that would, no doubt, produce all sorts of new sensations? I considered the research possibilities for five days. Finally, on the sixth day of class, I stopped by the lab after hours and took a quantity home to my room. After double-locking the door and parking my car around the corner in case anyone thought to drop by, I lay down on the sofa and began smoking.

While the thrill seeker in me was busily smoking, the scientist/detective in me was taking copious notes about my reactions. I described in detail the feelings I had: flushing in the head, tingling of the scalp and tightness in the chest. I felt that I could conquer anybody and anything. I experienced other sensations that were apparently unique to smoking cannabis. But as these receded, there was one other feeling that I couldn't shake: the feeling that I had done something quite wrong. I did not get much sleep that night.

On the seventh day, there were a number of bleary-eyed students filling the seats of the pharmacology class. The instructor began by pointing to the bowl of cannabis on the shelf.

"That bowl was full at the start of the term, just a week ago," he said. "It is now nearly empty, and I know why." He went on to say that he knew that many had participated in this act of curious clinical investigation. He then surprised us by announcing that he was undertaking a government-sponsored research project. He wanted to know, objectively, how smoking cannabis affected medical students who were bright, capable of giving a good history and able to describe their symptoms. He promised that there would be no repercussions for any illegality incurred during our "research."

I volunteered. I was particularly proud that I had kept written notes; only two others in our class had done so. We opened our notebooks and shared our scientific observations with the class. At the conclusion of our presentations, the instructor thanked us.

"Now, I have something to tell you. That bowl contained not a shred of cannabis. It was 100 percent Prince Albert smoking tobacco. I'm afraid your well-recorded sensations were all in your imagination."

The lesson so thoroughly taught by the instructor was, of course, the power of the mind, as well as the potent medicine of placebos. I was too amazed to be embarrassed at my gullibility. I have since made sure that those magic pills—placebos—are always part of my black bag.

I loved lab exercises in medical school. They were my chance to indulge my passion for detective work to the hilt. But there was one lab in our sophomore year that threatened to run away without me.

The experiment was designed to demonstrate the symptoms and treatment effects of thyroid disease. We students were to take vital statistics—such as pulse, respiratory rate and other measures of metabolism—of a laboratory rat, then sacrifice the animal and study the tissues. The exercise called for performing a thyroidectomy, or removal of the thyroid gland, after all of the data had been obtained.

My lab partner and I disagreed considerably over the proper technique to use in the thyroidectomy. I must have been right, because three of his rats died after his procedure, and after we had spent a lot of time getting their basic metabolic data. (He failed the task, left medical school and, I believe, is a very successful businessman today.) In any case, I still needed to pass this course, but since each of our rats had died, we could not complete our assignment.

Then I had an idea: radioactive isotopes were just beginning to be used in treating hyperthyroidism, or an over-reactive thyroid gland. I thought that if we could give the rat radioactive iodine to destroy the gland, we would have a live subject from which we could continue getting a metabolic evaluation.

But I forgot one thing: there would be no scars or marks on the rat's neck. There were hundreds of rats in the cage, and they all looked alike. How could we identify our rat in a cage full of many other rats that had not had surgery?

Then I had another idea: I could use a Geiger counter to determine which of the rats had been heavily exposed to radiation. I borrowed a hand Geiger counter and came back late that night. I stretched out under the cage, pointing the Geiger counter upward, and after a very long time I finally isolated the rat. At that moment, a group of my classmates walked into the lab. Imagine their surprise when they saw me under the cage. Imagine the awkward explanations, the hilarity, the whispers in the hallway the next day. One classmate recently told me that this was the only thing he remembered from his sophomore year of medical school.

In medical school I learned how to extract every bit of information I could about the patient in the time we had together, but I never had enough time to know the patient as well as I would have liked. I learned how to use the tools of my trade—the stethoscope, the otoscope and all of the other scopes available—but I learned quickly that my eyes and ears were my most important "scopes." I also used many of the complex instruments and the array of laboratory studies that were becoming available to the modern physician. I saw the importance of learning the history of medicine, which teaches us through discoveries of the past to be alert to unexpected clues given reluctantly and only for a very fleeting amount of time. Those are the clues that will lead to medical discoveries of the future.

No physician, young or old, believes that all of those marvelous medical discoveries are due to the brilliant planning of the scientific profession. Most of what passes for planning is really the result of serendipity, or discovery by chance. There are plenty of examples in history. It's a good thing for all of us that Dr. Joseph Lister observed the destruction of a bacterial mess in the city drains when carbolic acid was thrown in as a cleansing agent. And a good thing when the agar molds in Dr. Alexander Fleming's laboratory were contaminated by some escaped fungus material, floating up the stairway from the allergy laboratory on a lower floor. This led to the discovery of penicillin.

Planned reasoning, on the other hand, led Dr. Fredrick Banting, an orthopedic surgeon, after a sleepless night, to think through the currently known information about diabetes and to reason out the treatment by insulin of this disease. The same type of planned reasoning was used in the discovery of the cause of AIDS.

There have been serendipitous discoveries and planned discoveries; the physician must be aware of both. But during my years of practicing medicine I have seen certain serendipitous situations occur that have made major advances in medical knowledge.

As a sophomore student in bacteriology, I was asked the question that has been asked of medical students for over a hundred years. Toward the end of the Civil War, deaths from amputation, the most common surgical procedure, were much greater in the North than in the South, even though the surgical technique was the same. Why?

Supplies of foodstuffs and medications were considerably worse in the South due to the naval blockade. In the North, there were factories, better agricultural production and generally a superior ability to outfit the troops with the needed materials to maintain health. Scientists and medical professionals looking at these facts would assume that the North would have a far better survival rate from amputations, but that was not the case.

The answer, when we realized it, was very simple. The Northern blockade effectively prevented any imported goods from entering the Southern states. One of those imported items, which probably seemed dispensable at the time, was silk thread. Confederate army doctors needed something else with which to suture wounds, and a common substitute was horsehair, which was quite strong, but kinky. In order to straighten it out, it was necessary to boil it. Without knowing it, Southern surgeons were sterilizing their equipment, with the resultant dramatic saving of lives. It took almost a hundred years for this mystery to be solved and, like the discovery of insulin, the answer was found by reasoning. We don't know who solved this mystery, but the information continues to be helpful. Now researchers consider sociology and history in understanding disease (for example, in the relationship of homosexual behavior to HIV). As a young doctor, I became more and more appreciative of the largess bequeathed me by my predecessors in medicine. Down the road, it would inspire me to make my own contributions.

It is a cliché (but like many clichés, it's true) that doctors hold their patients' lives in their hands. It is a great responsibility, one that has become heavier in recent years, with new medications that either help or harm depending upon the side effects of the drug given. Furthermore, medications have so many potential side effects that the physician must keep constantly abreast of all new drug interactions. The proliferation of new drugs with potential for harm may explain why pharmacy bills are high, why research and development of drugs are so expensive and why approval of apparently useful drugs seems endlessly delayed. It means that every effort should be made to prevent errors.

I learned this lesson while I was a sophomore medical student. We were asked to solve a very complex medication problem. The correct answer depended upon knowing a number of detailed clinical facts and converting these facts into a proper dosage for the patient, involving rather simple arithmetic but quite a few mathematical steps. The difficult part was obtaining all the clinical facts. I spent days gathering the facts before I finally turned in my paper. It was returned to me with the ignominious grade of zero.

I was very upset. There were as many as a hundred facts necessary to solve this rather complex puzzle, and I had done everything correctly—except that I had misplaced a decimal point. That was just a simple mathematical error, I thought.

I obviously knew all of the other facts because I came to the right answer, with the exception of the decimal point.

I went, in some agitation, to see the professor. He looked me straight in the eye and said, "Mr. Banov, you are absolutely correct. You did all of these steps correctly. You knew a complex amount of information, and you did a splendid job. There is only one problem. Were this a real clinical situation, you would have just killed the patient by giving him ten times the dosage that he should have received."

That lesson helped me prepare vaccines and extracts for people with allergic problems. In immunology, picking up the wrong bottle could result in a mistake of 1,000, 10,000 or 100,000 times the dosage. We tell our students that they might make an error and give two antibiotics one day instead of one, or three or maybe four. But there is no way they would be stupid enough to give 4,000 or 400,000 times the dose. Or is there? All they'd have to do is make one mathematical decimal point error, and the patient dies. They get the point. Constant attention to the possibility of making a decimal point error keeps us continuously on our toes.

In medical school, lessons about respect for the human body apparently needed periodic reinforcement. This we received in our junior year, during training in physical diagnosis. In the obstetrics clinics, for example, it was the fashion for students to wear the bloodiest shoes and socks possible. This meant that the wearer had been up all night studying and could not spare the time for sleep or a change of clothing.

Far worse was the insensitive attitude of the male students when approaching a female patient for a pelvic examination. Rough, cold, gloved hands and an unsympathetic attitude were the order of the day. There was no one to correct the eighty medical students in our class—no one but the female students, who had already suffered from the tasteless jokes and inappropriate humor of their male classmates during the past three years. Three years, it turned out, was plenty of time to plot their revenge.

Medical students and physicians in training at all levels make bets continuously about every possible subject—for example, whether a certain lazy professor would again reuse a previous exam rather than write a new one. Our two female classmates, newly minted junior medical students with starched white coats, had acquired a few IOUs from bets lost by their classmates. Now it was payback time.

At one weekend party, while enjoying a bit too much wine, a few male students promised that we would repay our debts to the female trainees. This seemed safe enough. After all, how bad could the payback be? We soon found out.

Recently returned from the gynecology rotation, they wanted us to see how it felt to be on a cold examining table with some indifferent, gum-chewing male examiners probing and prodding. Although I prefer to forget the details, I do remember the fear that these gals inspired in us as we went through the "experiment." Our female classmates taught us a lesson in respect for the patient that has lasted a lifetime. The experience made a big impression on me and I asked (and the other students followed my lead) to be allowed to swallow gastric tubes, have intravenous lines inserted and even have a rectal exam—the ultimate in male indignity—so that we would be able to truly empathize with the patient. I now insist that all of my students and residents in training, when possible, try to experience some of the procedures commonly done on patients. It has certainly made all of us more caring physicians.

In his entire career, a physician never feels as knowledgeable and self-confident as he does at his medical school graduation.

But that feeling dissipates with amazing speed. I remember entering Milwaukee County Hospital on my first day as a brand-new medical intern, with my starched white coat containing not one crease. As I walked confidently into the ward, I saw a group of nursing students gathered around the charge nurse. They were in the midst of a training session. The nurse instructor asked if the students might watch my first procedure, which, I was informed to my shock, involved removing the patient's eye.

While I knew a little anatomy of the eye from studying *Gray's Anatomy*, I'd had very little experience with ophthalmology. Removal of the eye was a bit out of my league as a fresh intern. Fortunately, the nurse instructor was quite accustomed to interns. My startled expression alerted her that I needed an explanation. The eye in question was artificial; they wanted to see me remove it from the patient so that routine nursing hygiene could be performed. This prospect was even more frightening to me, as I had absolutely no idea how to remove a glass eye. I think I may have seen an ophthalmologic surgical procedure from a far distant room or in an amphitheater, but that is about as far as it went. I was surrounded by a dozen or more nurses and, as I was to discover many times during my intern year, there was no way to escape. I took a deep breath, stepped forward and put my hands on the patient's eyelid. The prosthetic eye popped right out into my hand, and I smiled as if I had been doing this for years.

This was almost as humbling an experience as my first obstetrical delivery. That time I forgot to put on my rubber gloves. The senior nurse gave me a small slap on the hand, which is something I never expected. As a doctor, I thought I had authority over the nursing staff. But here, I realized, was a very experienced nurse who was truly in charge, who knew she was in charge and would always be in charge, in spite of the hundreds of young interns and residents passing through her hospital. My realization was another necessary, if deflating, rite of passage. But it's never too soon for a young physician to learn that he or she is part of a team, and all the members of the team make valuable contributions. Sometimes that means knocking the self-important physician down to size.

Sometimes the students knew more than the experts. During rounds with our senior professor at the hospital one day, we passed a patient sitting in the hall who had some type of undiagnosed neurological problem. It seemed as if every specialist as far as Chicago had been asked to review this patient's case, and no one had any inkling what the problem was.

One of the medical students accompanying us on rounds was a nun who had traveled extensively for the church before going to medical school. As we walked by the patient, she commented, "Oh, I haven't seen a case of leprosy like that since I left Hawaii."

Although we had been studying this patient for many weeks and consulted many specialists, it took this student less than five seconds to make the diagnosis of tubercular leprosy. This was a good lesson. Healthcare workers have varying degrees of experiences and those individual bits of information make each person having contact with an ill patient a different reference source. So the more opinions we get or the more consultations obtained on a difficult diagnostic case, the more likely we are to find the correct solution. Much of the success of medical treatment depends on the luck of a physician to have experienced certain rare conditions and the ability to apply this experience to a patient perhaps years later. I have observed that the physician who is too proud to get a second, third or even fourth opinion when needed is not acting in the patient's best interest. I would not feel comfortable having such a doctor for myself or my family. In this case, we all benefited by the expertise of a medical student and that wonderful healing agent known as "tincture of good luck."

I met Nancy Leopold, the woman who would become my wife, in Milwaukee a few days after I arrived for my internship. I like to tell anyone who will listen that I met her in a mental hospital. Sometimes I say I picked up her name and telephone number in a public men's room. Take your pick. Both stories are accurate.

The first night I arrived in Milwaukee, I was apprehensive and homesick. My newly minted medical degree did little to reassure me when I realized that I knew a lot of theory but less practical medicine than a Boy Scout completing a first aid course. I decided to boost my self-esteem through the magic of Hollywood, and went off to see a corny, "doctor-as-God" movie—*Not as a Stranger*.

While in the men's room, I overheard the conversation of someone on the wall-mounted telephone. The conversation, from the one side I heard, suggested that the speaker was either a medical student or a physician in training, like me. After introducing myself, I learned that he was a senior medical student at the University of Wisconsin—and Jewish! What an opportunity to make my parents happy! I explained that I didn't know anyone in Milwaukee, had little free time and a list of available young Jewish women would be the ultimate act of professional courtesy.

My new acquaintance obliged me. On that list was a pre-med, med-technologist and graduate of the University of Wisconsin, who was working at a nearby mental hospital laboratory while going to classes to fulfill the medical school requirements. She lived at home with her parents, so I could have some expectation of invitations to dinner. He also correctly recalled that she was very good-looking. Her lab was closer to me than the location of any of the others on the list, and I was then, as now, interested in saving time. I walked over, and fifty years later, here we are. I can say I owe my marriage and the existence of my children to a full bladder. Actually, I owe only our first meeting to a full bladder: I got married because a top underworld boss made me an offer I couldn't refuse.

I miss the good old days, when organized crime ruled the streets of our major cities, but nurses, doctors and medical students were able to walk through the most dangerous, crime-ridden areas of the city to and from their hospital work, regardless of the hour or condition of the roads. It was out of bounds to rob them or harm them in any way. Nurses in particular were always protected and had no fear on their way home or to a bus. After all, a criminal could be their next patient in the emergency room. Now, with narcotic addicts and amateur criminals out on the streets, all bets are off, and the hospital worker walking home after a late shift had better beware. Organized crime at least maintained a standard of decency.

I was introduced to my underworld patron during my rotation in the emergency room. One evening during my shift, a nationally known gangster from the Fazio family was brought in. This very dapper gentleman had been drinking wine straight from the bottle; there must have been a chip in the glass, and he somehow had cut himself under his tongue. The small laceration produced a frightening amount of bleeding. He was taken to an emergency room where, because of all the blood, coupled with the patient's panic, the examining doctor was unable to find the bleeding source and simply had the patient go home with a bit of gauze in the mouth as a pressure dressing. However, the man's bleeding persisted, and he was finally brought to my emergency room about two hours after the injury. By that time, the blood in the cut had clotted somewhat, and I was able to put in one single stitch, which immediately stopped the bleeding. This required no great medical or surgical skill, but to the gangster's associates, who had accompanied him to the emergency room (and, in fact, all the way into the examining room), I had performed the most brilliant surgery of all time. They told me so many times over.

I chuckled a bit about this and then forgot all about the incident until a week later, when a frightening group of the most gangster-like characters I'd ever seen strode into the hospital, demanding to see the doctor who had operated on their boss. They were not ushered in to my examining room; they simply tumbled in, gathered around me and all but lifted me in the air. The ER staff was terrified, and I was beginning to worry a bit too, but they explained to me that the boss wanted me as his guest at a famous underworld restaurant at five o'clock sharp the following Thursday evening. I was to bring my "woman," or "girl," with me. It never occurred to me to say no. I doubt it would have occurred to anyone in that situation.

The only person approximating "my woman" at that time was Nancy, though I'd only had two dates with her. She was a good sport and accepted the date, even though she knew that our hosts, the Fazios, were big-time gangsters and there was no telling what we were in for. I didn't let her know it then, but I had no one else to ask. I think she assumed that to be the case, and she went along to protect me. She has been doing that now for over fifty years.

We arrived at the restaurant at exactly five o'clock. No other guests were present; there were only employees, all of whom looked like gangsters. (After my two emergency-room meetings with gangsters, not to mention numerous Hollywood movies, I felt sure I could identify a real gangster on the spot.) There were a few people assigned solely to our needs for this dinner. We were shown into a large, austere room with an extremely long table. It was a very dramatic setting for a fairly simple dinner for three. We were seated at one end of this vast piece of furniture. Arrayed in front of us were no fewer than ten varieties of liqueurs and before-dinner drinks, and we were invited to help ourselves by the boss, who sat a distance off at the far end of the table.

Neither Nancy nor I were experienced drinkers, and we began to feel the effects of all this alcohol very quickly. Once again, it never crossed my mind to decline his invitation to sample the booze. We only prayed that we would not do something foolish, such as choose a "sissy" drink. We tried to be careful, but by the time the meal came, we were drunk. Throughout the meal, the boss, my grateful patient, never said a word. He simply stared at us while drumming his fingers on the table in a very deliberate, and frankly scary, way. Eventually, the meal ended. We left the restaurant, almost unconscious from all the alcohol. We found a local movie theater where we could sit in the balcony all by ourselves and sober up for a few hours before we dared take a city bus back to the hospital. Not only was this a real bonding experience for Nancy and me, but it also definitely hastened our trip to the altar. After all, when a hardened criminal and local mob boss tells you that he likes your friend and is looking forward to her being a member of the family, he means it, and you listen!

My year in Milwaukee was lucky for me in more than one way. I met Nancy there, and my good friend Julian Atkinson interned in Milwaukee and roomed with me. Julian had one peculiar characteristic: an unusual type of sleep amnesia. If he should be awakened from sleep for a period of time at night, by the next day he would have completely forgotten any events that may have taken place. This was something that could be a serious problem for a practicing physician, even though we used to laugh about it in medical school. It certainly caused a serious problem for me on one occasion.

I had gone out with my future wife on one of our rare dates—rare because one thing that interns never have enough of is time. In my attempt to have a social life at the same time as a successful internship, I would often double date on one of the few evenings that I had off from hospital work.

Double dates to most people means two couples going out together, but for an intern or medical resident, a double date meant two different dates, one early and one late, in the same evening. All of this was managed on a maximum of three or four hours of sleep per night.

My late date that night was with Nancy. Our car got stuck on a dirt road. Believe me when I tell you that she was safe with me on that country road. She couldn't have had more security for her virtue than being my second-shift date after I'd gone thirty-six hours without sleep. In fact, she was quite safe from everything except my falling asleep at an inopportune time.

The car was firmly entrenched in the mud and we were forced to hike about three miles to the nearest store to get help. I spent my month's salary on a cab to take us back to the city.

After dropping off Nancy, I went back to the hospital and woke up Julian to ask if I might borrow his car to help get my car out of the mud. He got up, crossed the room to his bureau, retrieved the keys for me and wished me good luck.

The next morning, he awoke and was getting ready to go to an outlying clinic for a pathology conference when he could not find his car keys. When he realized his car was missing, he called the police and reported it stolen. The police issued a bulletin about this stolen vehicle, which, of course, I was driving. It didn't take long for them to pull me over. I explained to the police officer that I was an intern at the county hospital and that I had permission from my roommate to take his car. The police officer looked at me—disheveled, unshaven and distraught—and thought it might be wise to verify this situation.

The hospital director's office paged Julian. Some police officers wanted to ask him a few questions.

Had he given permission for anyone to use his car? Julian did not remember a thing about the previous night. In fact, he tried to help my case (I think) by adding that in his opinion I was too much of a nerd to ever get a girl to go parking with me on a country road. This information was radioed back to the local substation, where I was being held, to the amusement of my captors.

The hospital director had to come down in person to bail me out. I was subjected to his sarcastic comments throughout the year. In the end, being noticed, for whatever reason, was a good thing for me. I was the only intern he could actually remember over the next several years. That meant I could always be assured of a reference letter when I needed one. And in spite of my record as a car thief, it was always a positive recommendation.

Twelve months later, my internship was completed. Since there was still a military draft, I had to repay my medical school deferment and spend two years in uniform. I had two options: be drafted into the army as a buck private, or enlist as an officer and physician in the navy medical corps. Needless to say, the choice was easy to make. To a Southerner born and raised in a port city, the navy looked appealing. As it turned out, and with what's known as military logic, I never saw the ocean in my two years, and the only ship I saw was in a maritime museum.

Meanwhile, Nancy and I spent all of our free time together. One day we realized that we enjoyed being with each other so much that we never wanted to say goodnight. We never discussed marriage, we just drifted into it. I do recall being in the middle of a movie a week before our formal wedding when Nancy leaned over and reminded me that I had never asked her to marry me. I said that she was absolutely correct and I would do so at the end of the movie. Well, we forgot again. Now, fifty years later, with four children, six grandchildren and thousands of wonderful memories, we still do not like to say goodnight.

So a few weeks later we packed all of our belongings and set off for the adventure of life. Packing was easy in those days: we simply threw everything we owned into the car. Even loaded, it still had plenty of room to spare. As we drove away from Milwaukee, I promised Nancy one thing: she would never be bored. I do believe I have kept that promise.

Chapter 3

You're in the Navy Now

I completed my Milwaukee internship in 1956. The Korean conflict had ended in 1953, but two years of required military service were still a rite of passage for most young men. Without the threat of war, the thought of two years as a real doctor in the military was quite exciting. Fortunately, most of the military patients were in good health, with only occasional bouts of trauma and obvious diseases, such as appendicitis or gonorrhea.

Since this was essentially the first time any of us had any free time since high school, it was a treat to be in a situation where little academic pressure was placed upon us. We were not career officers, so we felt free to laugh at the military, with all of its glaring deficiencies and inefficiencies. The concept that we might have to march, dress uniformly and respect our ranking superiors with such ridiculous body movements as a salute, or by saying "Yes, Sir" and "No, Sir," was difficult for us to accept. We kept continuous smirks on our faces whenever any military duties were required. We were vastly amused at the idea that we had to dress up in our formal navy uniforms for inspection every few weeks.

You could spot a medical or dental officer in a large room or on parade because he just didn't look as if he belonged there. The professional officers barely tolerated the doctors. We were simply excused from anything military whenever possible. But it wasn't always possible.

We were commissioned as ensigns in the navy at a one-day orientation at the Great Lakes Naval Training Station in North Chicago. As soon as we completed the orientation and reported for active duty, we were automatically promoted to lieutenant junior grade. And, at the time I was inducted, physicians who had completed their internships were admitted as full lieutenants. Just before lunch on orientation day, we were told to get our uniforms and were given vouchers for that purpose. Everyone in our class got up to leave, except me. The chief petty officer, who I thought was an admiral because of all of the stripes on his arm, asked me why I was not going along with the group. I said, "Sir, I came into this navy as a lowly ensign at about eight this morning, and by noon I've gone up two ranks. I figure if things go on this way, I should be a rear admiral by sundown." I explained that it didn't make sense to buy my uniforms until I got my stripes straightened out. Apparently this instructor didn't think my comments were as humorous as I did, because he quickly got my attitude straightened out.

I was sent to the U.S. Naval Air Station at Beeville, Texas. This was a center for training naval and marine jet aviators and ground crews bound for carrier duty. It was very exciting to think that I was about to play a role I'd only seen in my imagination. It was somewhat deflating to be told, along with all the other medical officers, not to hitch rides on the planes. The orders were, "This is an advanced air training command. Don't get in the way."

Getting in the way turned out to be a big temptation, because we were not very busy at the base. Sick call was from 8:00 to 8:30 a.m. After that, we seemed to be free all day long. The navy periodically evaluated its need for physicians, and noted that our station had too many doctors for its very few patients. But every time an inspection team came by to verify this, more doctors were sent to the base.

We were bored. Well, not entirely bored, as Nancy gave birth on December 8, 1957, to our first child, Mark Samuel Banov, in Corpus Christi. But concerning military and medical action, there was not much going on in the middle of Texas during peacetime, with no real enemies around. The Russians didn't seem concerned with destroying Beeville.

One day, the boredom was interrupted by a knock on my office door. A young officer came in and handed me a sealed envelope marked "Secret." My heart raced, but I was prepared. I had been given a directive about what to do when we received a secret document. The protocol was to go to a secure location, read the information and hand it to another officer. I assumed the document was of major importance because the young officer who delivered it wore a large handgun. The only secure place I could find in my office was the bathroom, so I went in, locked the door, sat on the john and opened the envelope.

The top-secret document said, "This is to inform you that as of this date, all U.S. Navy aircraft carriers will have atomic weaponry available." This information was to be shared with no one and not discussed among military personnel. Of course, the first thing I did was go home and tell Nancy. She realized that this was probably not a very serious situation, but she reminded me that if I did not want to risk a court-martial I should probably follow the directions. For three or four days I enjoyed a secret bond with the physicists who developed the atomic bomb, as well as with every spy from Mata Hari to the Rosenbergs. My bubble burst the next Saturday night, when we went out to a movie. There on the newsstand was the cover of *Life*, stating that all U.S. carriers would soon have retaliatory nuclear potential.

So much for military secrets.

Our long periods of boredom were interrupted by the adrenaline-stimulating sound of an alarm telling us that one of our training jets had crashed. The doctor on duty stopped whatever he was doing and ran to the back door of the dispensary. Within minutes, a rescue helicopter arrived, hovering a few hundred feet overhead, dragging a rope and sling. The doctor grabbed the rope and was pulled into the rapidly ascending helicopter. At the crash scene, the doctor was lowered to the ground by the same rope.

I was terrified each time I was pulled through the air on that rope. Making it into the helicopter didn't calm my fear: we only had to get out again, this time in midair, and be lowered by the rope to the injured pilot. I am not a particularly courageous person, and it really upset me that my colleagues, who were as timid as I, seemed to enjoy this ride! After my last rescue mission and another harrowing flight through the air, I was returning to my office and conducting my usual search for dry pants. My chief petty officer, Chief Neely, knocked on the door.

"Hey, Doc," he said. "I been meaning to ask you something. Why do you always get into that sling backward? You're gonna get yourself killed like that!"

Was it an oversight that no one, in two years, had seen fit to inform me that the sling was for the arms and shoulders, not the feet? Why the hell didn't someone tell me that all I needed was to put the sling under my armpits to enjoy the ride like everyone else? Had I been overheard glibly remarking that we didn't need any training to be navy doctors? I guess I didn't know it all, after all.

The Beeville station's clinic had a very elaborate set of operating rooms and trauma rooms, as well as numerous sets of the most up-to-date and expensive surgical instruments. Yet almost every patient requiring a surgical procedure, from an ingrown toenail to an appendectomy, was sent to the naval hospital at Corpus Christi, about sixty miles away.

However, the navy, in its wisdom, decreed that one surgical procedure could and should be done at the local facility: adult male circumcision. You might think this would be a rare request, but in the navy it provided the patient with an automatic thirty-day leave after the procedure. That, plus the misconception that circumcision prevents venereal disease, resulted in thirty-three beds of our thirty-four-bed ward dedicated to post-circumcision recovery cases.

I remember that ward well. All the beds were in a neat row, with a nursing station visible and accessible to all of the beds. At the nursing station was the chief nurse, an obese, stern, commanding officer–type civilian who made certain that everyone knew she was the boss. There was really only one big nursing responsibility for these patients: to immediately administer an ethyl-chloride spray to prevent the obvious complications of a normal healthy male's erection, should it occur before the sutures healed. As soon as one of the patients had an urge to elevate the bed sheet, he simply raised his hand and the nurse ran over and gave him a squirt of ethyl chloride, a local anesthetic agent that was very, very cold. A cold squirt on the discomfort of a fresh circumcision caused the sailors to exclaim, "The flag came down from the flagpole."

If nothing else, the underutilized physicians were provided with opportunities to perform surgery, but I doubt that any of the doctors who served during that time ever wrote in their curriculum vitae that they were extremely experienced at circumcision and no other surgical procedure at all.

Navy physicians did encounter one major problem in the late 1950s: patients did not respect the dangers of venereal disease. Penicillin had been around for a few years, and the most common disease, gonorrhea, was so easily treated with a single shot that sailors drove down to Mexico and returned almost every month with a fresh case. Eventually, urethritis, or chronic urinary tract problems, awaited these young men. Illustrated pamphlets and frightening movies on the effects of VD were no help at all in getting the sailors to protect themselves. We were facing a true epidemic.

So we designed all sorts of techniques to impress upon the patients the dangers of their irresponsible actions. One that was most effective we called the "New Treatment Routine." I had heard of this from one of my senior hospital corpsmen, who knew more about venereal disease than any medical authority in the military. After an intransigent young man came in with his fourth or fifth case of gonorrhea, we called him into a windowless room. One physician indicated that, unfortunately, this time he had contracted the Korean variety of gonorrhea, which was unresponsive to all medications. The physician sorrowfully explained that amputation was the only method available for preventing the spread of this disease all over the body. We left the sailor alone for another hour to contemplate this news. Then a second physician on the team came in holding a medical journal. "Wait, wait!" he shouted. "No amputation, no amputation. There is now a new treatment! That is, if nothing is done, there is no need for amputation because within three weeks it will just fall off!" Not one patient, after receiving the New Treatment Routine, ever returned with a repeat case of venereal disease during the rest of my stint in the navy.

I did have an educated senior officer call me at one o'clock in the morning to ask whether a certain variety of condom, which was made out of sheep gut, would be effective in preventing venereal disease. I sleepily told the officer that I did not know that information but that I would look it up first thing in the morning and let him know. He replied, "But, Doctor. I can't wait until morning to find out!"

Despite the opportunity to play soldier, I remained bored. I had worked long and hard to become a doctor and now I was stuck here for two years, with precious little outlet for my energy. Then I happened to drive through Pettus, Texas, one day. I don't know what benign spirit whispered to me to stop the car, but the decision to do so only took a second. If it had taken any longer, I would have been past the town and halfway to the next one. The entire town consisted of three commercial buildings: a gas station, general store and some type of geological business. But to the farmers in the area, Pettus was a metropolis. I met the keeper of the general store and my bright idea sprang from our casual conversation: I would open my first private practice in Pettus. Soon enough, I was installed on the second floor above the store.

Through the help of Chief Petty Officer Neely, my guardian and protector, I acquired some surplus materials from the base and outfitted my small office. Nancy and I cleared away the cobwebs and covered the large holes in the walls with free travel posters. The result was a dusty, dirty, unattractive, inefficient office, but it was my first real office, and Pettus's first doctor's office.

Medical specialists often look jealously at the old-fashioned country doctor, carrying a few magic potions in his little black bag; helping people when few options are available; totally responsible for the medical needs of a small group of patients, instead of dispensing expert advice for only one part of the patient. Modern medicine demands specialization, but specialists must surrender that marvelous mutual interaction that can develop between physician and patient in a family practice. Those months in Pettus showed me what it might have been like to be a country doctor, even though that kind of practice was soon to be a relic of an earlier age.

I especially remember my obstetrical experiences. In one instance, a woman in labor was brought in after a midwife had fought with a complicated delivery. The baby was in a horizontal position and absolutely stuck in place. The patient was severely dehydrated, and death was a strong probability for both mother and child. The semi-trained nurse, a former surgical assistant in San Antonio who had some formal X-ray training, felt that we must do a cesarean section. I had never performed a cesarean, though I had participated in them, and I was a product of the philosophy, "See one, do one, teach one." We did a section on this patient, and miraculously she survived. At least, a half-miracle occurred: the mother survived, but the baby did not.

I delivered four other children, and the deliveries were all uncomplicated, making me think I was really superfluous to the whole event. I performed my first unsupervised forceps delivery, which was a little scary even though everything went well. I received praise from the grandmother, who was an observer but probably had been present at more deliveries than many obstetricians in their first year or two in practice. I even assisted at the delivery of a litter of golden retriever puppies. I really had no idea how dogs are born, but nature is a good teacher and I didn't want to disappoint the anxious children watching me watch the dog. I decided not to tell them about my unusual birth and why I feel a special appreciation for veterinarian skills.

On another evening, I was preparing to leave the office at about ten o'clock at night when two very distraught young Hispanic men came up the stairs. They told me that their grandmother was dying and the family needed me immediately. I had no opportunity to offer any excuses or even ask where Grandmother was. One of the young men was closing the door for me, turning out the lights and guiding me very firmly by the arm out the door. Outside I saw two automobiles filled with more young men, all of whom appeared to be equally distraught. It looked like a caravan was about to take me to Grandmother. I had no time to call my wife and say that I would not be home, nor did I have the opportunity to take my own car, as I was handed into the back seat with two very burly, heavyset males on either side of me.

I truly wondered if I were being kidnapped. I was very careful to tell my escorts that I had no money with me, but they did not seem to be particularly interested in that. I spoke no Spanish, and that was the only language my captors knew.

After driving for many miles and a considerable time, we arrived at an isolated house where I saw other cars and members of the family in the yard. I was ushered into a bedroom where Grandmother lay in obvious heart failure, having great difficulty breathing. More family members surrounded her so closely that I feared there wasn't enough air for her to breathe. I wasn't sure what would come next, but my mind inevitably turned to my first great information resource: the movies. Hollywood had taught me that when kidnapped by thugs, you'd better save Grandma—or else. On the other hand, my medical training taught me that my patient had severe cardiac decomposition and would need advanced medical treatment—in a hospital—if she were to have any chance of recovery.

This was absolutely not acceptable to the family. If Grandmother were to die, she would die in her own bed. They were very firm in telling me that I should do everything possible to save her. For the next four hours I tried everything I could. I isolated the extremities with tourniquets to relieve the heart from circulating so much blood, gave mercurial diuretics (which were the best available at that time) and tried to open up the pulmonary veins. My black bag held one ampoule of a digitalis-type medication, which I used to try to regulate her heart rhythm.

But in spite of these attempts to save Grandmother, she died. I was prepared to be the human sacrifice to follow her, but this did not occur. What did occur was considerable wailing, crying and an outpouring of emotion that eventually was directed toward me—but in a positive way. With the greatest appreciation at having witnessed medical science's best attempts at saving a life, family members hugged me, patted my back and had me go over and kiss Grandmother (which was apparently a mark of respect). I have never felt so venerated and appreciated as I did at that moment.

The young men escorted me back to the car, drove me back to my office and said goodnight, with many more thanks.

I felt ashamed of my earlier fears. Just because these folks did not speak my language and were from a different culture, I'd assumed that they would not understand my attempts to save this woman's life. While I was silently praying for her recovery, I was really praying for myself. What I had felt was most immature and unfounded. But what I had done was what a real doctor would do in spite of personal fear.

In Pettus, I learned what it meant to be a doctor.

My Pettus medical practice made my two-year navy stint pass a lot faster. But there were plenty of medical officers for whom the Beeville posting was permanent. Our chief medical officer, Dr. Frank, was in his early fifties when I was there. He wasn't a very impressive figure: obsequious with the naval officers to whom he reported, stuck at a dead-end south Texas station, terrified that he would be cut from the service even though he was a Korean conflict veteran. We younger physicians didn't have much respect for Dr. Frank, or for other medical officers who, like him, had to maintain both military and medical lives in order to survive.

But one day I fell into conversation with a couple of older officers, veterans of the 1950 Inchon invasion. They told me about a medical officer who had been a hero at Inchon, spurring his fellow soldiers on, remaining with the wounded until they were stable, never thinking of his own safety. The doctor under discussion turned out to be our unimpressive and obsequious Dr. Frank. He himself never told us stories about those battles, and from his behavior we never would have guessed.

That day I realized that heroes come in many styles. In fact, the more time I spent in the navy, the more I lost my cynical, cavalier attitude toward the military. A fighting machine could not be expected to be efficient in peacetime. A combat-ready jet on an aircraft carrier is a waste—until it is needed. We learned to respect and admire the professional pilots, no older than we were, who were dying in crashes while we watched reruns of *Victory at Sea*.

One evening, when the student pilots were playing volleyball in front of the medical building, my senior corpsman called me at home and told me that some of the students were messing with the X-ray equipment. Since this obviously could be dangerous, I immediately came down to the base and found one of the students in the building, closely examining a wet X-ray film that he clearly had just shot and developed. I angrily explained to him that X-ray equipment was dangerous to the untrained operator, and there was no reason for him to be using it.

He led me into another room and quietly explained that he was, in fact, a fully trained flight surgeon stationed in New Orleans, whose job was to go through classes along with the student pilots, posing as a student himself. He could then get an inside glimpse of what life was like for them and if the training programs were good or bad, proper or improper.

What an effective method of obtaining information! Or, perhaps, what a great storyteller! I never found out which he was.

Aside from my fellow medical officers, I had the most contact on the base with the petty officers. They were superbly trained, confident (though sometimes a bit too confident) and very protective of a young physician.

One day I was called into the kitchen, where a group of the corpsmen with whom I worked asked if they might have a little talk with me. Young medical officers were generally called in to see the petty officers, and not the other way around, as the higher-ranking physicians were dependent on the seasoned, enlisted hospital corpsmen.

The first week I was in Beeville, the corpsmen tested me by suggesting a different treatment than the one I had recommended for a patient's rash. I recognized the corpsmen's concerns, and made a seventy-mile trip to Corpus Christi to buy a very large dermatology text, which I used for a detailed lecture on rashes. I explained to the corpsmen that I was in charge of the medical problems and they were to do all the navy stuff—rank be damned. At no time would we compromise or allow compromise on patient care. Providing the textbook for their study was a major compliment to them and earned me their acceptance.

The men with whom I worked liked me. In fact, they liked me so much they wanted to be certain that I had some hobbies that they felt would be important in my future medical career. They offered to take me dove hunting.

I had never hunted and did not wish to hunt. In Judaism, it is ordained that one only eat animals that are ritually and painlessly slaughtered. Also, one should not kill animals except for food. But these fellows were determined, and when they are in command and you are a young, inexperienced doctor, you'd better listen and listen well. Petty officers issue orders that traditionally can take precedence over those of the admiral.

I tried to be a good sport, but after six months I had fired off numerous shotgun shells and never once hit a dove. Finally, the same group of petty officers called another conference.

"Doc, you're just not a hunter," they said. "No matter how hard we try, you're never going to be a hunter. It's lucky that none of us got killed. But since you're a nice guy, we decided to chip in and buy you some golf lessons. Most doctors play golf, and we're sure you'll want to join a country club and play golf."

After never hitting a dove in six months, I took my first golf lesson and struck a beautiful drive down the fairway. Unfortunately, there was a dove in the way, and I hit it. After that, I gave up both hunting and golf.

The 1950s was an important period in the navy's aviation history. The rudimentary jet airplanes, first used in combat in Korea, were now being improved, with sophisticated, state-of-the-art electronics. But some problems still resisted solution.

One was that when a pilot had to eject from the aircraft in an emergency situation, the abandonment of the plane occurred at an altitude of well over fifteen thousand feet. Supplementary oxygen was provided from a small tank strapped to the pilot's leg. After making the decision to eject, he had to remember to disengage the small oxygen tank from the large central one. He also had to blow off the canopy of his seat before ejecting.

In addition, the pilot needed to wait until his altitude was about ten thousand feet before deploying his parachute. If he did not wait, he would descend too slowly, run out of oxygen and possibly lose consciousness. So the pilot had to free-fall with his parachute closed for a period of time determined by his height and weight. When the appropriate time elapsed, the pilot would pull his ripcord.

As if all of these tasks were not enough, there was another problem. In those days, the pilot sat on his parachute. After the entire ejection seat, with the pilot strapped to it, was blown out of the aircraft by a piece of TNT, the pilot had to release his seatbelt so his chair could be discarded and the parachute could open. These pilots were the most intelligent, best trained and most physically fit officers in the navy. And yet the pilots often became confused and were unable to open their parachutes. They pulled on the ripcord while still sitting on the chutes. They would be found miles away from the crash site, their bodies broken and distorted, seat belts clawed and ragged. In their desperation to open their parachutes, the pilots forgot that they were sitting on them and until their seat belts were released the chutes would not open. If they were wounded in flight and lost blood, they would be more likely to make a mistake.

In Korea, pilots often sustained severe injuries to their upper and lower extremities. The protocol was to attach a small length of rubber tubing to the dashboard of the cockpit with a rubber band. Holding one end of the tubing between his teeth, the injured pilot could apply a very rudimentary tourniquet so that he would not bleed to death before all of the necessary escape maneuvers could be affected. Unfortunately, in the process of being blown into the air at considerable pressure, the tourniquet could easily be dislodged, and the pilot would begin bleeding again, possibly going into shock and eventually losing consciousness.

One day I was discussing this problem with Nancy, who was a teacher and medical technologist. I was discouraged at learning about the loss of two pilots in a single day. Both lives could have been saved if they'd had a more sophisticated, tourniquet-like device. Nancy offered a brilliant idea: if pilots wore antigravity suits, perhaps the pressure in the suit could create a complete tourniquet.

She suggested putting a small release valve in the arms and legs of the G-suit. Then when an injury occurred, the pilot could simply deflate the suit except for that portion above the injury. This is similar to what is done on submarines when damage is sustained to the vessel: certain compartments are sealed off. We took home some flight suits and Nancy made a prototype on her sewing machine. We sent it off to the Bureau of Medicine and Surgery of the navy. For months we heard nothing, until one day an officer with a little briefcase came to visit. He congratulated us on inventing something that was very much needed. He told us that the suit would be researched and tested in certain divisions in the navy.

We never heard another word about it for twenty-two years. Then, one day in Charleston, I was giving a physical examination to a senior naval officer. He told me that his responsibility for the last few years had been research and development.

"This is a long shot," I said, "but have you heard of the device my wife made?" I described the invention to him. He told me that he had been working on the very same project for quite some time. It was used in the American armed forces for a number of years and then sold to South American countries, where the suits were in use for many years more. I like to imagine how many lives Nancy's excellent idea—not to mention her ability to operate a sewing machine—have saved.

In the early 1980s I received a routine letter from the U.S. Naval Hospital stating that all physicians who were consultants to the military and not on active duty would require periodic updating of their credentials and applications. Soon a multi-page form arrived that I was to ask a colleague to fill out, attesting to my good character and competent medical skills.

I received this on a busy morning and refused to fill out this piece of bureaucratic silliness. Furthermore, I was a bit embarrassed, at that stage in my career, to ask my colleagues to testify as to my good moral character and the fact that I was probably not a child molester or rapist. I thought it would be more dignified if I simply had one of my friends in medicine complete the form. I chose Dr. David Arno, a close friend and colleague who had been on active duty in the navy for many years before going into private practice in orthopedics. When he mailed it back to me the next day, I handed it, unread, to one of my clerical workers. She submitted it to the appropriate office of the navy. The day after, I received another envelope from Dr. Arno containing the same completed application.

Realizing that I had received it the day before, I asked my transcriptionist if she had, by any chance, made a copy of that earlier application for our files. She had. When I took a look at it, I was shocked. The first application contained answers to questions such as, "How well do you know Dr. Banov?"

Dr. Arno's answer: I've known him well over the years and have had to apologize for him on many occasions.

Question: Do you know anything about his ethical and moral background that could be injurious to his career as a consultant at the Naval Hospital?

Answer: If I can't say anything good, I'd rather not say anything at all, but there are things that were just not up to snuff.

Question: Do you know of any lawsuits or medical-legal problems currently being investigated and ongoing?

Answer: Well, I understand via the grapevine that there are many problems. You really have to check with Dr. Banov on this.

And so on. The second application was completely different, including all the nice things that one would say about a colleague. When I told Dr. Arno that I had not looked at the first form but had simply mailed it on to the Bureau of Medicine and Surgery in Washington, he was aghast. He had meant this as a joke. He was sure that I would read the first application and call him.

It was a tremendous practical joke, but it had backfired. I was indignant. I ranted and made a fuss. I insisted that Dr.

Arno stop his work, reschedule his patients for the day, call Washington, work through the layers of bureaucracy and tell the folks in charge it was all a joke.

This he did. The chief admiral, under whose watch this particular credentialing took place, came to the phone and chewed him out. He said that this was the United States Navy, not a bar where practical jokes were tolerated. He would report this to his superiors, and Dr. Arno could be assured that legal action would be taken. The admiral advised Dr. Arno to contact his attorneys.

What Dr. Arno never knew is that before calling him, I called Washington myself. I explained to the young medical officer with whom I spoke that this unfortunate incident was a practical joke gone sour. He agreed to help me turn the tables on my friend. We arranged for Dr. Arno to receive a cold reception, a stern lecture about submitting false documents and a warning about the likelihood of government wrath.

The naval officers involved told me they had the greatest laughs of their careers.

Chapter 4

Training to Be a Real Doctor

My two years in the navy lasted a lifetime, or so it seemed. At the end, I left Texas a more experienced general physician, but with some important decisions to make.

First, I needed more training. The age of specialization had begun and it was becoming evident that a young physician would no longer be able to do it all. Even though legally the state's license granted me the authority to practice medicine and surgery, modern urban hospitals required appropriate residency training in order to have admitting privileges. There was even talk of postgraduate certification for the family doctor or general practitioner. Great progress in medical research was making it impossible for even the most astute physician to keep up and be fully knowledgeable in all phases of medicine.

The problem was that I liked it all. I needed to choose a field that would give me the intellectual stimulation and satisfaction of diagnostic and therapeutic challenges. At the same time, I wanted a specialty that would allow me to assume the role of a family physician and provide for the nonsurgical needs of my patients.

The field of internal medicine was the logical choice. However, I felt that I was making a tremendous concession in becoming an internist. I would be giving up the thrill of delivering babies and taking care of children, and I'd miss out on the ego boost of being the "god in white" of surgery. I looked for a teaching hospital where I could be exposed to the greatest variety of patients as well as good teaching facilities.

I found what I was looking for in 1958, when I walked into the monstrous, three-thousand-bed Charity Hospital in New Orleans, to begin a residency in internal medicine. Charity Hospital was one of the most unusual facilities in the country. It had provided medical services, often free of charge, to patients on all rungs of the socioeconomic ladder since the 1920s. It was built, along with other charity hospitals, by the infamous and corrupt governor of Louisiana, Huey Long. Charity was one of the good results of Long's stormy, dictatorial leadership of the state. Two medical schools shared this behemoth, and were located on each side of the hospital. The facility was so large that two residents at the same hospital could go to Tulane or LSU medical schools and never run into each other in their four years of training. Charity Hospital survived many physical, legal and economic crises over the years, but Hurricane Katrina was too strong an adversary; the beloved old giant took water damage from the levees and the gunshots of looters until it just rolled over and closed its doors.

What I remember about my days at Charity are the interesting and inspiring teachers, more than the facts they taught us. I remember the patients' personalities and their concerns. I observed how they adjusted to their illnesses. Some of the more difficult and less compliant patients were so demanding that staff, caretakers and often their physicians rejected them and they received even less attention; they were always unhappy and lonely. These patients, I found, were really depressed and frightened. They had the most difficulty communicating and needed more attention and understanding than the passive patients, who simply accepted their illnesses without resistance. I could see that the art of medicine was to be able to win the confidence of the patient, no matter how grave the diagnosis might be. I found that what patients needed most was for people to care. When the young physician realized that, caring became natural, and the real physician was born. From then on, science and humanity worked together in harmony, with the physician being the conductor. That's what I learned and remember most, and I pray that those lessons will never be forgotten.

I learned so much more from listening to my patients than from textbooks and medical journals. The famous medical teacher Dr. William Osler, from Johns Hopkins, once said, "Listen to your patient, he is telling you his diagnosis." He said this in the early twentieth century, before CAT scans and MRIs. I teach my students to organize their approach to a patient by following this firm rule in any situation: first, the patient; second, the patient; third, the patient; but always, the patient.

On a rainy late afternoon in my second year of residency at Charity, I saw my last patient of the day, a seventy-year-old Cajun woman from the bayous of Louisiana. She had the distinction of having been in the Charity Hospital system all of her life. She had grown up there, delivered her babies there and received whatever other medical care she needed over the years in that same old, uncomfortable, crowded medical clinic. This lady had what she called a big problem. In the late 1950s, oil was discovered in some of the bayous, and those who, like my patient, owned land there could lease the oil rights for large sums of money. She would gain significant income for the first time in her life, but this made her ineligible for the medical services of Charity Hospital. She needed to choose a physician in the community to take care of her.

There were hundreds of Charity-trained residents who practiced in the New Orleans area. My patient had contact with many physicians over the years, and we all wondered who she would choose as her family physician. After all, she knew from firsthand experience who the best real doctor was.

Speculation ran high for weeks. Finally she chose a man who practiced on the periphery of the city, although it was inconvenient for her to go out to his office. I was quite surprised at her choice. This man was a perfectly acceptable physician, but he was certainly not someone with "Best Doctor of the Year" potential. In fact, he was one of the blandest and least exciting residents I had ever worked with—I even thought him rather lazy. How had she come to choose him? I couldn't suppress my curiosity any longer, so I asked her how she had made her choice.

"You know, Doctor," she said without hesitation, "I have seen many, many doctors over the years—as a little child, a grown mother and now as an old lady. In all those years, this man is the only one who helped me put on my coat."

In all the years and of all the doctors, only one had thought to extend that courtesy to her. It was clear to me that she had made the right choice.

As a second-year resident in medicine at Charity, I had the traditional benefit of accompanying the famous Dr. Edgar Hull, who was chief of medicine at Louisiana State University School of Medicine, on his annual visit to Carville for his consultations on cardiovascular problems in the leper colony there. Carville was one of the only leper colonies still in existence in the United States, and it was always fascinating to go there and see numerous patients in the presence of a revered medical teacher. But Dr. Hull was also very savvy about medical politics and how to get his programs accredited and funded at a time when there was stiff competition for federal support of medical teaching hospitals.

A few days after our Carville trip, Dr. Hull and I entered a hospital elevator along with one of the inspectors from the Joint Commission for Accreditation of Hospitals. As we were riding up, Dr. Hull commented that his hospital should be accredited because the residents had such extensive clinical experience.

"For example," he said, "here's one of our residents. Dr. Banov, how many cases of leprosy have you seen as a medical resident in the last week?"

Of course, "the last week" included my visit to the leprosarium a few days before, so I said, "Last week I saw, oh, at least twenty-five cases of leprosy."

"Thank you very much, Doctor," Dr. Hull replied, then got off the elevator (rather quickly, I thought) at his floor.

I do not think any further inspection was necessary at the hospital after it was reported that this training program was the best in the world because the physicians had such excellent opportunities for study.

Dr. Edgar Hull was an extraordinary teacher. He could do more, diagnostically, with a stethoscope than modern cardiologists can ever begin to do with all of their sophisticated equipment. When Dr. Hull made his rounds in the morning and pointed out heart murmurs, he had as many as twenty-five physicians following him, just to hear one or two beeps from his stethoscope. His ears were magic and his touch the quintessence of diagnostic sensitivity. He co-authored one of the original books on electrocardiography and always elected to remain as a medical school professor rather than accept the many offers he received for lucrative private cardiology practice.

He once attended a medical meeting in Nevada and became ill. He was treated in an ER facility by a young family practitioner whose potential was evident to Dr. Hull's keen eye. He invited this young man to come back to Charity Hospital and train in internal medicine. This physician, whose expenses were all paid by Dr. Hull and his family, became a leading teacher and practitioner of geriatric medicine. He achieved national and international accolades for his teaching and practice.

In the early 1980s, pharmaceutical companies and medical professors realized that no one had heard anything about or from Dr. Hull for several years. He seemed to have disappeared. The staff of *Modern Medicine*, one of the popular medical journals of the day, took on the task of locating the famous medical teacher and cardiac researcher. They found him doing family medicine in the bayous of Louisiana. He was working twelve hours a day, delivering babies at home and, in general, handling an extremely difficult practice.

The searchers asked Dr. Hull if he had financial problems, or some difficulty in his family. Perhaps he was ill and needed funds for extra medical care? His reply was very simple: all of his life, he told them, he'd wanted to be a country doctor and practice good, solid medicine. Events led him to become a medical school teacher, and before long he had many responsibilities, nationally and internationally, in medical education. But he was undeterred from eventually achieving his dream.

To me he was another true example of a real doctor.

There aren't many Charity Hospital trainees, besides me, who would list Dr. Walton R. Akenhead among the more interesting and influential teachers of their medical career. He rarely officiated on grand rounds, although he made many significant remarks and generally arrived at the correct diagnosis. Dr. Akenhead is not remembered at all in the scientific community outside of LSU and Charity Hospital because he did not subscribe to the "publish or perish" principle. He once told me that in the time he might spend preparing a publishable paper, he could see any number of sick patients, not to mention do more of what he loved most—teaching.

Dr. Akenhead had two major dislikes in medicine—one was stuck-up Ivy Leaguers, and the other was the science of statistics. He often emphasized that in statistics, if the odds were one in one million, for one patient statistics just didn't matter.

One memorable grand rounds session was chaired by a visiting professor who won the Akenhead jackpot: he was a stuck-up Ivy Leaguer giving a boring lecture on statistics. No one understood the lecturer, but only Dr. Akenhead would admit it. It so happened that the visiting professor was quite tall, about six feet five inches. At the conclusion of the lecture, he asked if there were any questions. No one responded except Dr. Akenhead, who exclaimed, "Doctor, I don't like or understand statistics, but I do know one thing: according to statistics, you should be five feet eight inches tall, and if that is the case, why you wearing them long pants?"

Dr. Akenhead had just made another of his marvelous clinical diagnoses in a way that only he could do, and he made it to an audience that will remember well the lesson and the man. He insisted that we appreciate each patient as an individual, unique and independent from the faceless and indistinguishable disease statistic. This is why I get upset when I hear a student or house officer ask me to see a lung abscess or a sinusitis in Bed Four. Dr. Akenhead would have retorted, "No, Doctor, there is a *patient* with a lung abscess in Bed Four."

It was Dr. Akenhead who witnessed my patient having the symptoms of paroxysmal cold hemoglobinuria, which led to my first published article in a medical journal. Here was a classic example of serendipity. There is a hematological condition in which the patient has red-colored urine after exposure to cold conditions. The color is due to hemoglobin, a part of the blood, which has separated from the blood cells and is then expelled from the body. It is a very frightening and embarrassing experience for the patient. It's thought of as one of those many diseases that medical students learn in school but never see.

When I was the on-call resident in medicine at Charity, a patient was admitted one night for pneumonia. While I was in the course of taking his detailed history, the patient described to me a classic case of paroxysmal cold hemoglobinuria, but he said that he was now cured of the disease. Even at three o'clock in the morning this information caught my attention. With the rare exception of associated syphilis, I remembered that this blood condition was untreatable and certainly not curable.

I continued asking about his past history and learned that he had had an automobile accident some years before, and had ruptured his spleen. The organ was removed. After that, no more paroxysmal cold hemoglobinuria. Interestingly and quite by chance, Dr. Akenhead had witnessed the patient having grossly discolored urine prior to his automobile accident. Both the patient and Dr. Akenhead were at a family wedding some years before, and Dr. Akenhead noted the discoloration of the bowl after they both had used the toilet. He advised the patient to consult his personal physician and he recalled some annoyance and resistance at this unsolicited advice, especially since the patient was feeling quite well and had not seen his doctor in over five years.

I could not wait until the morning for the medical library to open. A literature search showed that a splenectomy, although used to treat other blood conditions, had never been tried for this condition.

I published this information as a clinical note in the *Journal of the American Medical Association*. It appeared in two pages way at the back of the journal. However, I had requests for reprints from all over the world. I had unintentionally discovered a possible treatment for an incurable condition. In addition, the information led to the further investigation of the immune properties of the spleen, and indicated a new direction for immunological research. I sent a reprint of the article to one of my mentors at the Medical College of South Carolina. His comment meant so much to me: "Well, Charles, you've just repaid your debt to those of us who educated you. The rest will be profit." Thanks, Dr. Vince Moseley of blessed memory. I hope your investment has paid a good premium.

During our orientation session on the first day of my residency at Charity, I met another new trainee, Dr. John Salvaggio. He was a Cajun Italian who had never been away from New Orleans. He reminded me of my good friend Julian Atkinson from South Carolina, but there was something about John, a look or a manner, that made me believe he would make a significant contribution in medicine.

John Salvaggio viewed each patient's medical situation as a mystery to be solved, and also as an important research statistic, one that might eventually lead to a cure for disease. He had that twinkle in his eye when he had an idea about a disease, an intellectual curiosity that itself was contagious. He spread it immediately to anyone who observed him at work.

John and I saw many patients together, but we approached the same patient in different ways. I would worry about the disease's influence on the patient, and John would look at the disease as a scientific challenge. Since we were both intending to sub-specialize in allergy and immunology, we spent hours discussing the merits of private practice medicine versus academic university care and research.

John Salvaggio became a professor of medicine at Tulane, as well as a prolific researcher in the field of allergy and immunology. I went into private practice, but not before helping John get out of New Orleans for a time, and into his future career.

There was no doubt about it: the residency was hard, and I was always thoroughly exhausted by being on call every other night and portions of most weekends. Although my fellow residents and I complained constantly, we realized that the busier we were and the more responsibility for patient care we had, the more we would learn. It has been axiomatic for years that the better teaching hospitals work their residents more, pay them less, respect them less, feed them less and permit them to sleep less. In the end, those are the most desired residencies. Survivors of those programs spend the rest of their lives complaining to their families, colleagues and patients about how they suffered, how they were merely cheap labor for the hospital. And they are partly correct: it is only now, in the twenty-first century, that monitors of physician training have realized that perhaps the patients for whom these tired house officers minister suffer as a consequence.

In the 1950s, the conventional wisdom was that long hours with resultant sleep deprivation make a better doctor. But too many incorrect doses of medication are given or surgical errors are made by a conscientious resident trying to extract maximum learning from every minute of his residency period. I learned a great deal while at Charity—and the hospital got a great deal out of me for fifty dollars a month.

Obviously, one could not support a family on fifty dollars a month, even in the 1950s. For the physicians this meant either moonlighting and doing some out-of-the-hospital practice on the weekends, or borrowing from family, a demeaning action for a thirty-year-old son who had been subsidized most of his life. I did both.

While walking one evening in the French Quarter, my wife and I had an idea: we would hire a babysitter and Nancy would join the group of sidewalk artists doing portraits and caricatures. She'd always had a talent for painting and we were sure she had infinitely more talent than the artists we observed.

There was only one problem: she needed a license. This was no big deal in most places, but in 1958 New Orleans, a significant number of the "artists" truly did not have painting talent. They were quite successful in more horizontal skills.

The city was just beginning to enforce their anti-prostitution ordinances. In order to obtain a license to paint in the French Quarter, it was necessary to provide a document stating that you were not a prostitute.

My wife refused to ask her friends to provide such a document. That left only my parents to vouch for her. Nancy simply would not ask her new in-laws to state that their daughter-in-law was a virtuous woman. I guess I can say without exaggeration that my wife could not help with the family expenses because she could not prove that she wasn't a prostitute.

It was during my residency in internal medicine that I found myself drawn to the subspecialty of allergy and immunology. At that time, it was one of the newest, and perhaps smallest, fields of focus. In 1960 there were very few truly great training centers in the subspecialty of allergy. It was a significant achievement to be selected as one of two fellows at the Massachusetts General Hospital Allergy Training Unit under Dr. Francis C. Lowell.

Even so, upon arriving in Boston I felt as if I were a young child on the first day of a new school. I was irritated at myself for feeling anxious. After all, I had spent four years in college, four years in medical school, a year in a rotating internship and two years as an internal medicine resident. All that, plus two years as a physician in the navy, should have given me some degree of confidence. It didn't! The profession of medicine seems to demand of its members the continuous presence of self-doubt and constant self-assessment. I realized this decades later, when one of my sons, after a grueling medical school exam, asked me when it was that I felt I really knew enough to consider myself a good doctor. I replied, "Not yet."

My first hurdle was to find an affordable apartment for my family, now grown by the addition of our first daughter, Lori Lynn Banov, on August 4, 1959. Nancy and the two children were staying in Milwaukee with her parents while I apartment hunted. At the same time, I needed to extract every opportunity from my fellowship, which meant spending as much time as possible in the hospital—day and night. To me, this second imperative meant that I need not find a place to stay during my first weeks alone in Boston. I would do what I'd done before.

In the past I had learned that I could find out about hospitals and training programs by traveling and sleeping during the day and wandering about the wards and chart desks at night, hearing the comments and complaints of the staff. I recalled my good fortune in my first week in Milwaukee, when a chance meeting with a medical student in a men's room netted me the telephone number of an attractive medical technologist who became my wife. This time, however, I was a staff member (even if one step lower than the assistant janitor) of the most famous hospital in the world. The physicians' lounge might serve as my networking center and hotel room.

At good old Charity Hospital in New Orleans, it had been perfectly acceptable to plop into any vacant bed in the physicians' lounge. It was most certainly not acceptable at Harvard's august Mass. General. Since I didn't know that, I plopped, uninvited, into an empty bed belonging to the chief resident, Dr. K. Frank Austen.

Dr. Austen was the only physician I've ever met who was so outstanding that he passed his board examinations while still in training. A world-class researcher and professor of medicine, Dr. Austen was president of our American Academy of Allergy and the International Association of Allergy and Clinical Immunology.

He was a bit surprised to find a stranger in his bed, especially since senior residents at Mass. General were not known for logging much sleep when on call. He was a gentleman about it though, and elected to find another place to sleep. The problem was that I didn't find an apartment for my family for a week, and I'm not certain what Dr. Austen did for that time. He was probably out looking for a hit man to take care of me. He never mentioned the subject during the entire year I was in Boston and I thought he'd forgotten about the stolen bed.

Years later though, I had a problem, almost a Catch-22: I was unable to obtain a formal endorsement of my character, integrity or ability from any board-certified physicians or Fellows of the American Academy of Allergy—not because I was disreputable, dishonest or incompetent, but because there were no other persons in my state (or in the neighboring states) who were themselves certified. Without the endorsement, I could not take the allergy subspecialty examination. Without the examination, I could not become certified!

I finally wrote to Dr. Austen, reminding him of our year together at Mass. General and keeping my fingers crossed that he would remember only my first-rate medical work and not our awkward introduction across the rumpled bedsheets of the physicians' lounge. His reply both reassured and unnerved me: "How could I forget you? You stole my bed!"

Dr. Austen wrote my recommendation, declining to brand me an uncouth bed thief, and as a result I was able to become one of the first and only certified allergists in the Charleston area.

The Boston physicians were so impressive and dignified that it was a big surprise, on that first day, to recognize a familiar face from my medical school days in Charleston: Dr. Andrews, who had made such an impression on my parents when he came to dinner one Friday night with his friends, the chimps. After medical school I hadn't seen or heard from him until that encounter in the lobby of Mass. General. I asked him about the chimps, but something in his answer made me ask no further questions. I never saw Dr. Andrews again.

It was not until I returned to Charleston to practice that I found out what had really happened. Dr. Andrews had accepted a two-year grant to allow his chimps to live in his world, observing them to see if neurological changes occurred. According to the grant proposal, after extensive neurological testing with the primitive electroencephalography available at the time, he was then to sacrifice them. He couldn't do it. Dr. Andrews might have lost his scientific credibility, but not his loyalty to his best, and probably only, friends.

The chief of the Allergy Training Unit, Dr. Francis C. Lowell, was of the famous Massachusetts Lowells. If ever there were regal Americans, the Lowells would be classified as such. They were high society. There was no greater social achievement than to be invited to the home of a Lowell.

Francis C. Lowell could have been a spoiled aristocrat; instead, he became one of the most respected immunological researchers in the world. He fine-tuned the double-blind technique of scientific inquiry, whereby any medical therapy could be evaluated accurately for its effectiveness. Medical science did not know then, nor do we know now, the answer to many disease treatment mysteries, but through Dr. Lowell's efforts we do have the techniques to determine whether something is true or not. That is crucial after so many useless treatments over the years. Fortunately, Dr. Lowell's work preceded the AIDS and SARS epidemics, and his techniques of evaluating treatment programs have made major contributions to world health.

Dr. Lowell was never impressed with his heritage, and people smiled behind his back about the Lowells not talking to

the Cabots and the Cabots talking only to God. Yet Dr. Lowell
was a true gentleman, with impeccable dress, superb manners
and an adolescent innocence about how the rest of the world
lived. I recall that when John F. Kennedy was elected to the
presidency, I asked Dr. Lowell if he had visited the Kennedys,
since they lived quite near each other at Hyannis Port. One
of Dr. Lowell's other colleagues told me I had embarrassed
Dr. Lowell when I asked that question, because it would be
unthinkable for the Lowells to have any social connection
with the Irish Catholic Kennedys. Nevertheless, one could
find every possible color and creed—a true American melting
pot—in Dr. Lowell's laboratory. Honesty in scientific research
was his sole criteria for a person's worth as a physician and
researcher.

After spending a year at patients' bedsides and in research
laboratories, I came to see that I did not have sufficient interest
in research to become a Dr. Lowell. I would have to make my
contributions in a less dramatic way. I had such respect for Dr.
Lowell that I often felt that if I were ever in armed combat
with my life threatened, Dr. Lowell could lead me anywhere.
He just had that charisma. Yet he could not lead me into
the path of research, despite trying very hard. Instead, my
personal contribution to the field of allergy and immunology
came when I introduced him to John Salvaggio.

I hadn't been in Boston more than a few weeks when I called
John, described the fascinating research being conducted in
our field and implored him to come up and join me. Most
die-hard New Orleans residents (and John was one if anyone
was) would never move even as far as Mississippi. Boston was
unthinkable. Nevertheless, John did come up to spend a few
days with me. I was able to make the intellectual marriage
between Dr. Lowell and Dr. Salvaggio that persisted until
both of their deaths a few years ago. They did fascinating
research together in Boston. Dr. Salvaggio took a three-year
fellowship with Dr. Lowell. There he learned the laboratory
and research techniques that enabled him to make major
contributions to understanding diseases of allergy and the

immune system. For example, he helped determine the cause of the New Orleans asthma crises, a condition that suddenly sent hundreds of people to local hospitals in just a few hours. Dr. Lowell is credited with determining one of the causes of diabetes treatment failures, among many other significant contributions.

John Salvaggio went back to New Orleans to build what became a very prominent career in academics and research. I became successful in private practice and gained some attention on a national and international level, but Dr. Salvaggio was one of the most sought-after lecturers and researchers in the world. Whenever I was on a program with him, I was fascinated by how much I learned just by being around him. But our private conversations were often about whether we made the right choices in our careers, because we started off together and took such divergent paths. He often expressed the wish that he could have earned more money in private practice for his growing family; I often wished I could make a greater contribution to the world. We two were clearly opposites but, just as clearly, had the same moral values and goals for our lives. In the scope of things, there has been room for both of us.

I knew I'd chosen the right specialty for me—one that involved a good bit of detective work—when one of the most interesting mysteries to occur in immunology was solved during my fellowship year.

All physicians and most laypeople knew that exposure to house dust could produce nasal congestion, sinusitis and even asthma. But the elements of house dust aren't usually very interesting or toxic—just assorted junk. Nevertheless, by giving tiny injections of house dust, allergists could help patients build up their resistance or immune response to dust.

At the clinic, we prepared injections using dust from two different sources. Both sources came from very reputable, FDA-controlled laboratories, but even using the same technique of extraction and preparation, the dust from one source was far more potent than the dust from the other source. Allergists had known this for years, but until one bright student thought to question it, no one asked why there was such a difference in strength. As with Lister, Banting, Fleming and other famous researchers, this student simply was not satisfied until he solved the mystery.

First, he discovered that both of the companies that supplied the dust had contracts with used furniture businesses. They used dust from old mattresses. But why would the mattresses from one company contain more potent house dust than from the other?

He delved further into the problem and found that the company with the most antigenic—most effectively potent—dust obtained its used mattresses from the red-light district of New Orleans. The other company, which had the less antigenic material, acquired its used mattresses from the Bowery flophouses of New York. We thought this an amusing but insignificant bit of information. But while we were snickering about the mattresses from the red-light district, our young inquiring scientist was asking another question: "What is so unique about house dust collected from mattresses?"

People are not allergic to house dust, but to the house dust mite, a microscopic organism that obtains its nutrition from human dandruff and skin flakes. Flakes from human bodies produce adequate food, and the more scales from the human body and the more dirt and debris, the more mites proliferate. The injections we were giving patients consisted of a small amount of mite and a good deal of nonspecific protein (the dust) that did nothing for the patient. So the dirtier the mattress, the more mites per ounce of dust; the more mites per ounce, the more potent the dust injections.

Again, when this information was presented, we all thought it amusing, but our inquiring student was not satisfied. It didn't make sense, he said: the occupant of a mattress in a Bowery flophouse must be far dirtier, filthier and therefore more mite-producing than the occupant of a mattress in a swanky New Orleans bordello. What was so unique about the red-light district's mattresses that made them such rich breeders of mites?

Our colleague would not rest until he found the reason: mites like different varieties of food, as do humans. The more variety in a restaurant, the more customers; the more types of human dander produced, the more mites. The ultimate difference between the mattresses from the Bowery and the mattresses of the red-light district was that there was only one body per night on the flophouse mattress and many bodies per night on the bordello mattress.

Recent studies have suggested another factor in the dust-allergy saga. There was a very high exposure of cat dander in the red-light district, as most of the inhabitants of that area owned cats, compared to the alcoholic homeless, who had no pets. Perhaps the cat exposure was also a factor in this mystery. It also suggests a possible derivation of the slang word for a house of prostitution—a cathouse.

Now that's research.

In 1960, I was peripherally involved in an incident that led to a breakthrough in our understanding of asthma and a certain kind of lung disease. An airliner had crashed on takeoff at Boston's Logan Airport. Investigators determined that a flock of starlings had been sucked into the jet intake of the plane, causing it to crash. One of the survivors was critically ill with inhaled jet fuel. The injured man was en route to a trauma center in central Boston, but dense traffic kept the ambulance from moving fast enough. The patient was almost dead from obstructed breathing. The ambulance attendants panicked and deposited their passenger at the first hospital they saw, which was Mass. General, not usually considered a trauma center. As the allergy fellow on call, I saw the patient when he came in. He was in severe respiratory distress. He seemed to be dying from asthma.

Not long before, cortisone had come into favor as almost a miracle drug. It was already used for so many diseases that the joke phrase "no one dies without cortisone" was practically an unwritten (and unscientific) principle. So for no acknowledged medical indication of the time, the patient was given an intravenous injection of cortisone—with dramatic results.

Up to that time, asthma was thought to be a disease of spasm of the breathing tubes. All of our therapy was directed toward relieving that spasm. We now know that there is also a strong inflammatory component to the illness. The spasm is only the trigger. Cortisone treatment addresses the inflammatory component of the disease.

Forty-five years later, while volunteering as a physician after Hurricane Katrina, I applied that knowledge. Hurricane victims were exposed to contaminated water from the broken levees. This time, we knew that the life-threatening component would be the inflammation produced by the water. We immediately administered high prophylactic dosages of the cortisone drugs and saved many lives. What a cycle—an airplane crash, an unplanned visit to the wrong hospital (which turned out to be the right hospital) and lives saved after a hurricane many decades later!

Chapter 5

Hanging up the Shingle

After my fellowship year in Boston, I decided to launch my medical practice in Charleston. My parents had never exerted any pressure on me to return, but I knew that nothing would make them happier than to have their son, the doctor, back in town. My mother was so excited that she went out and found an office for me near Hampton Park, in a less affluent part of town. Actually, it was part of a pharmacy on the ground floor, but with its own entrance.

My mother was a brilliant marketer. She thought it wouldn't look good for a young doctor to have his office in a pharmacy because it might seem as if he wasn't very busy, so she arranged to have the pharmacy repainted on the outside. Half of the exterior was one color, and the other half was a different color, which made it look like two separate establishments.

And, in a more personally embarrassing display of marketing genius, she kept the windowed front door uncovered. Without curtains or shades, her son, the doctor, would be visible to all her friends walking by. I remember also that she advised me not to accept cash payments from any of the patients that we knew, but to send them a bill. This way, she figured, they'd be reminded of my name when they saw it on the invoice. She suggested that while I was building my practice she could send over a few friends and relatives to sit in my waiting room so it would not seem so empty. I objected to that, but I do believe it was no coincidence that a few of her friends regularly dropped by during office hours to check my magazines for stray coupons.

Charleston in 1961 was slowly desegregating; one of the many ways it was changing from the city of my childhood. Of course, it was under various court orders since 1954 to do so, but real change doesn't happen overnight, especially in the South.

My kids simply don't believe me when I tell them what it had been like: the hospital had black male and black female surgery wards. Black and white pediatrics wards were standard, all in the same hospital, although then we called them colored, not black, wards. "Colored" was considered the more polite term. The local paper carried want ads for "colored" domestic help. Someone called the newspaper and asked, "What color?" The Department of Justice must have seen those ads too, because soon after that the ads dropped any mention of color.

For me, there was never any question that segregation—racial prejudice of any kind, in fact—was ridiculous. I remember observing my first operation in medical school. The surgeon made the first incision in the patient, who happened to be black, and as he bled I thought to myself that everybody should see an operation. Nowhere is it more literally demonstrated that everybody truly is the same beneath the skin.

But I was as inexperienced about racial issues as any other white person in Charleston. My parents had encouraged me to bring a "Negro" friend to dinner and couldn't understand that I didn't have one. How could I, since I'd always gone to segregated schools, and never shared a movie, or even a water fountain, with blacks? I'd known black workers who toiled in my parents' garden, and I had rewarded their labor with a glass of ice water that made me think of myself as a great liberal. I had no social relations with black persons of my age and had no black friends until long after medical school. Had I asked any of my black neighbors in the 1940s and '50s to come to my home, maybe to participate in a backyard ball game, they would have been equally as uncomfortable as I. College and medical school: still no black students. The best I could do for a minority friend in medical school was a dark-complexioned student who had been born in Laredo, Texas, with a cleft palate. To my provincial parents, he was my Hispanic friend with a Spanish accent.

Up at Mass. General, Bostonians chided me about prejudice in the South. But Charleston didn't have the kinds of riots that occurred up North in later years.

Still, breaking unwritten rules was not welcome. Charleston doctors treated both black patients and white patients, but the usual arrangement, still in practice in 1961, was to seat them in separate-but-equal waiting rooms. When I arrived, my office was one of the first, if not the first, to have a desegregated waiting room.

More than one colleague called to say that it was inappropriate for me, as a young person just starting my practice, to desegregate my waiting room. They warned that I would have a problem adjusting to the community if I made it known that I did not have two waiting rooms. I was proud of it, but at the same time somewhat intimidated by these disguised threats. I did need referrals, and I was concerned about losing patients. Then I had an interesting experience.

After 1964, when the doctrine of separate but equal became illegal, doctors still employed de facto segregation: they scheduled all the black patients for appointments on a certain day or a certain time period. If you were white and went to a doctor's office in Charleston for a scheduled appointment, you would see nothing but Caucasian patients in the waiting room. But if you happened to have an emergency and went in at a different time, the waiting room might be full of black patients. It was very quietly done, and the government didn't like it at all. To find out if doctors had this sort of de facto segregation, the government asked questions like, "How long does it take a black patient to get an appointment at your office, and how long for a white patient?"

My first office had come with a large partition down the middle of the waiting room so the previous tenant could claim it was "separate but equal." My family had the partition removed before I arrived in Charleston. Marketing was one thing, but there was no page in my mother's training manual for prejudice. "So, you have forgotten where we came from?" she would have said to me. "You think American slavery was bad—try lifting a few rocks for the Egyptian pharaohs!"

Fritz Hollings, at the time our ex-governor (later to become our very colorful U.S. senator for thirty-eight years), was my first celebrity patient. He was coming in for allergy testing, and I wanted to be sure my office made me look busy and successful. Naturally, my secretary scheduled him for the morning, when it was more likely that there would be a few patients in my waiting room.

Then it was I who had an emergency. Nancy experienced an ectopic pregnancy and needed surgery right away. Hollings had arranged to come all the way from Columbia to Charleston that same day, just to see me. It seemed I had to choose between my first celebrity case and my wife.

Nancy won, of course, which meant that I would see my distinguished patient after my wife's surgery was over, in the afternoon. At that time of day the waiting room held patients who had been going to the outpatient charity clinics (these were the days before Medicare and Medicaid). By the time Hollings walked in, the waiting room was filled with patients, all right—all working men, black and white, making minimum wage and on state medical aid.

Like most young doctors just starting off, I practiced de facto segregation—not by color, but by socioeconomic level. For those of us who had not yet built a reputation, the appearance of the waiting room and the patients was considered very important. Call it snobbery if you like, but that's the way it was. When I began practicing, a prominent older colleague told me that no one likes to dine in an empty restaurant—people assume the food must not be good. That's probably something they teach in business school for new restaurant owners. My mother certainly knew it, even without a graduate degree.

My celebrity patient was very gracious about the five-hour delay in his appointment. He sat in my waiting room with the other patients, reading, conversing and conferring with his aides. He even offered to let another patient—a mother with a few screaming children—go in ahead of him. I think he respected my decision to attend to my wife before my patients, and he could not have cared less about the environment of the waiting room or the skin color of the people waiting in it.

That day confirmed for me that it didn't make a bit of difference: all patients, famous or not, are equal in the waiting room and the examining room. I decided I didn't need to worry any longer about what certain doctors or patients might think. They would just have to get used to the arrangement I knew to be right. And the incident helped break the ice with Fritz.

I am certain most physicians cherish the memory of their first patients. I will never forget mine.

I was either the winner or first runner-up for the title of "Most Anxious Doctor Who Ever Lived." And although I was then a married man and a father, with years of schooling behind me, there was a lot I didn't know. For one thing, my Jewish upbringing had taught me nothing useful about other religions. So it stood to reason that the most anxious doctor who ever lived should be presented with a Roman Catholic nun for one of his first patients. The equally anxious young nun was brought into my office by her own chaperone, the mother superior of her convent. Her attention to her patient's viral sore throat easily could have earned her sainthood and a statue.

Nuns still wore traditional habits back then. Above a floor-length black tunic, a wimple and veil covered my patient's head, forehead and neck. Of course, I knew none of those terms at the time, but I assumed an air of lofty calmness. I casually said, "Now if you will just lift up your habit, we'll take a look."

The patient looked shocked. The mother superior stepped forward: "Doctor, surely you don't mean for her to lift up her dress simply to examine her throat?" Never in my years of medical school training had I ever learned the definition of a nun's habit.

That was only the first of many learning experiences for me as I dealt with not only my patients' symptoms but also their widely varying lifestyles. Medical school hadn't prepared me for these circumstances.

One of my patients, for example, was a well-known vice lord in the Charleston area. He was into prostitution, fencing of stolen goods and pornography distribution. His young daughter was one of my first pediatric allergy patients. She responded beautifully to treatment, and after about six months this businessman came to see me in the office.

"Doc," he said, "I know you have just started in practice here. I am sure you could use some help with the competition." He proffered the gift of one "job," meaning he would break arms or legs, threaten or perform whatever other services I asked on any of my enemies. I had one free ticket for this service. He carefully explained that my gift certificate did not cover heavy jobs such as "hits," which I assumed meant murder.

I thanked him politely. In the years that followed, there were, I admit, times when I considered how nice it would be to solve some problem by calling in my gift, but I always resisted the temptation.

After I was in practice for a few years, a colleague in a community near Charleston referred a patient to me with severe bronchial asthma. Her treatment was a success, and she was most appreciative. She made certain that we had numerous referrals from her place of business. We had not seen more than a handful of patients referred by her when we realized that she was the madam of a well-known motel/brothel near Georgetown, South Carolina. She just wanted to be certain that her girls got the best care.

C.

On Mother's Day in 1966, when our three children (Mark, Lori and Michael David Banov, who was born on September 3, 1962) were quite young and Nancy was very pregnant with our next child, we decided that for a special treat we would take a boat trip to a little community on the Intracoastal Waterway, about twenty miles down the river. We piled into our small boat along with my parents and one of the neighbor's children who asked to come along. We thought it might be unwise to have Nancy ride in the boat, so she drove down on her own and met us at the marina. There was a restaurant there, and we arranged to meet at the boat landing.

Nancy arrived a bit early and thought to herself that it was a lovely place. And wasn't it nice that they catered to cadets from The Citadel—she could see quite a few of them coming and going from the motel. Obviously, they must have been given a special rate, because most college students could not afford to stay in marina motels.

Before long we joined her and went to the dining room where, to our surprise, there were no other customers. We were seated at a table, but soon noticed that the waitresses were not very experienced. They seemed rather anxious, dropped a tray or two and never could get our orders straight.

The manager seemed extremely unhappy, not to say agitated. We felt sorry for him. After all, here it was a holiday afternoon and he had no customers at all, aside from our group. We assured him that we would tell all of our friends about the restaurant and see if we could help him build his business. This only seemed to make him more upset.

We had a lovely afternoon. We were halfway back to Charleston when it dawned on us what was really going on. Everyone in the small community knew what this motel's main business really was. Although the marina was a regular operation, it proved to be a good location for a brothel. The dining room was used almost exclusively for the workers there. When a happy family of grandparents, parents and children arrived for a nice Mother's Day dinner, some of the girls were pressed into service (and into uniforms!) as waitresses. The last thing that manager wanted was for us to spread the word about our wonderful dinner!

The next day I received two phone calls at work from patients of mine: "Doc, was I surprised to see you at the marina!" I jokingly replied that I, on the other hand, wasn't at all surprised to see my patients there. My fifty-eight-year-old father was even congratulated by a colleague, who had a boat in that marina, for having such interesting pastimes at his age.

Of course, many patients turn out to be not quite what they seem. I took care of an old gentleman for two decades whose appearance and actions told me that he had limited funds. Each time he came in for an appointment he brought me some produce from his farm: a few tomatoes, possibly a watermelon and occasionally some okra. He was probably one of the best-known and best-treated patients in our practice. There was a bond between us.

One day he brought his wife with him. She sat in the waiting room while I examined him. While he was undressing, I told his wife how touched I was that he always brought me a few pieces of fruit or vegetables in a little brown bag.

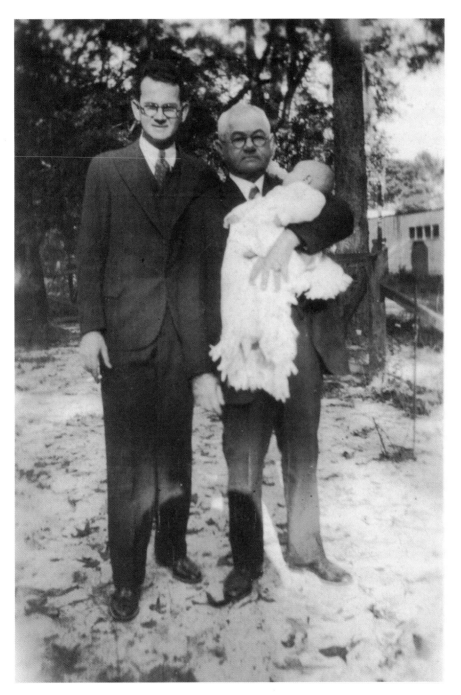

1. Three generations: my father Milton Banov, my grandfather Sam Banov (the unofficial Jewish doctor) and myself. 1930.

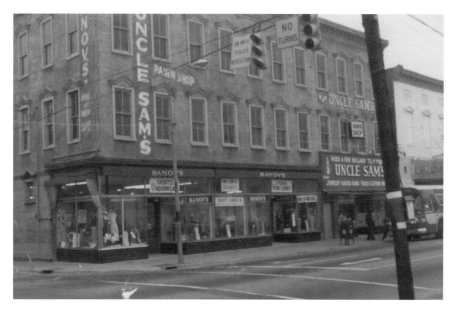

2. My grandfather founded Banov's Clothing Store in 1888. It survived a century, until it was destroyed by Hurricane Hugo in 1989. Here, in 1974, it was located at 595 King Street in Charleston.

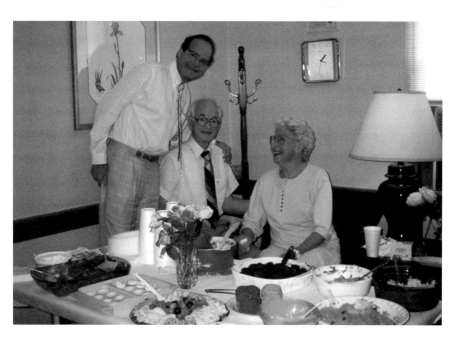

3. We were fortunate that my parents lived long enough to see their grandchildren grow to be responsible adults: my father Milton Banov until 1991, my mother Edna Ginsberg Banov until 2002. Here we are celebrating Mark's graduation from medical school.

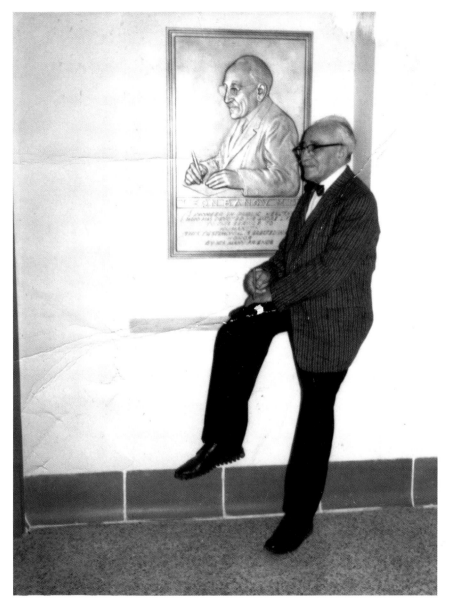

4. One of my heroes: my cousin, Dr. Leon Banov Sr., after whom the offices of the Charleston County Health Department were named.

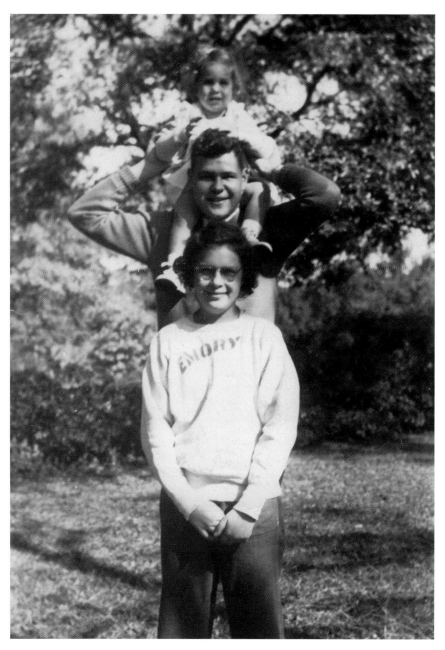

5. A Banov totem pole of Caren (top), Charles and Linda, 1948. Nine years separated each of us.

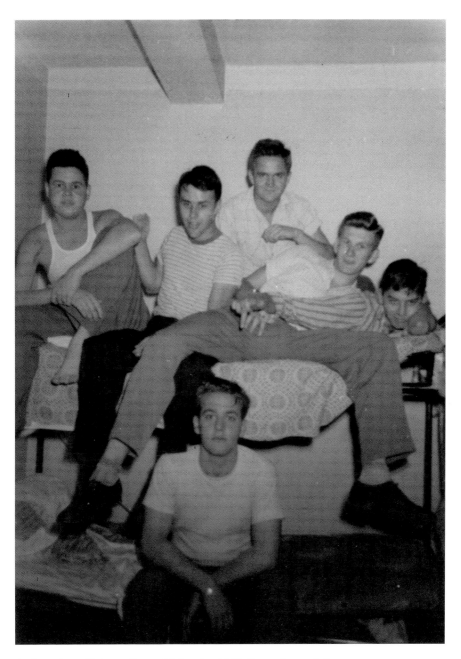

6. *Above:* A scruffy lot at Emory University, 1948. I'm at the top left.

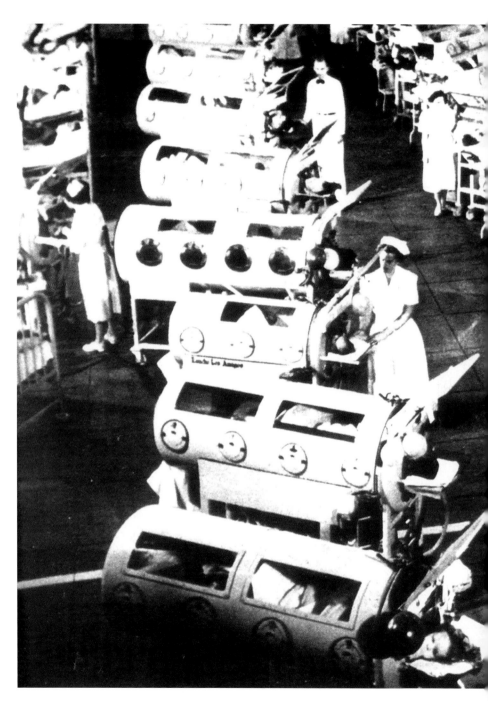

7. A common sight in the 1940s and 1950s: a roomful of "iron lungs" for children with paralytic polio. Recently I was surprised to learn that none of my office staff even knew what the machines were. Now that's progress! *Courtesy of Warren E. Collins, Inc., and nSpire Health.*

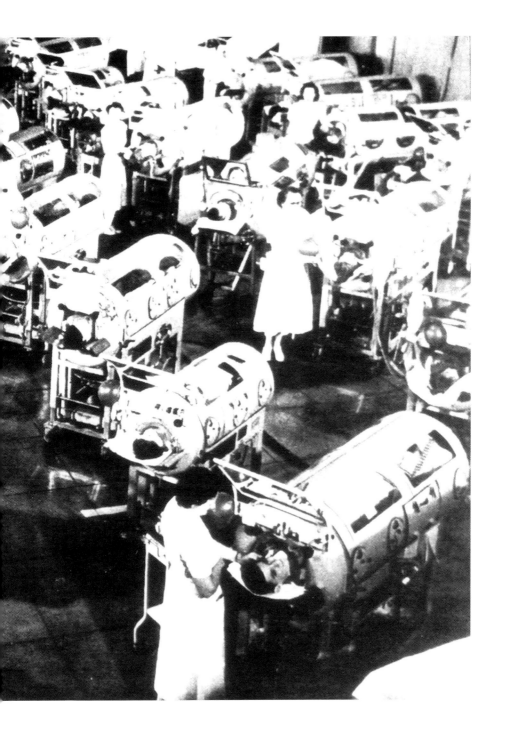

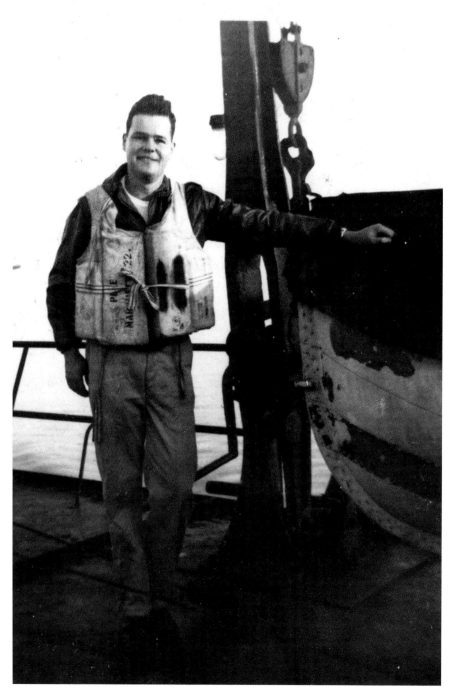

8. Between college and medical school, I signed on as a merchant marine, traveling to South America on an oil tanker. I had developed sufficient skills only to wipe oil from the engines and peel potatoes. June 1950.

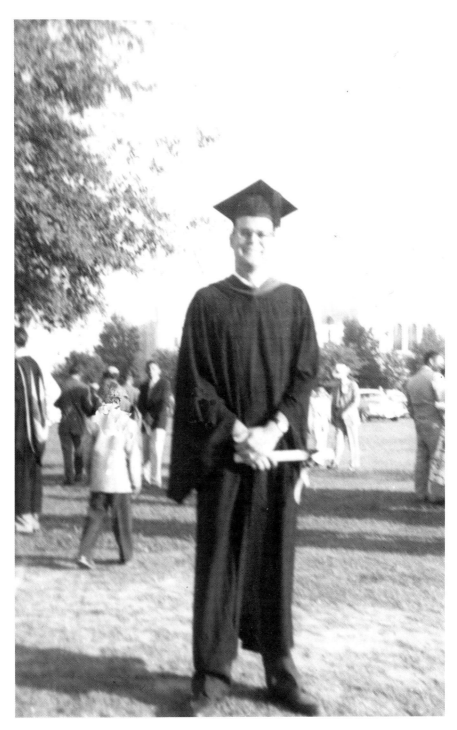

9. Graduation from the Medical College of South Carolina. 1955.

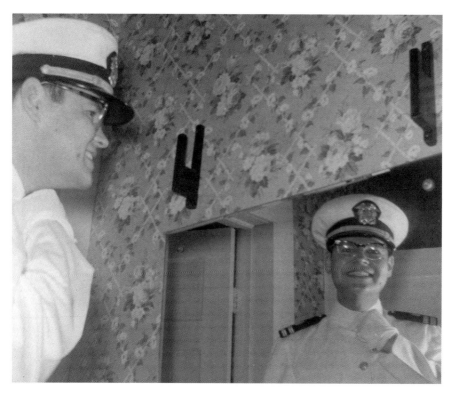

10. Proud to be wearing my navy whites. 1957.

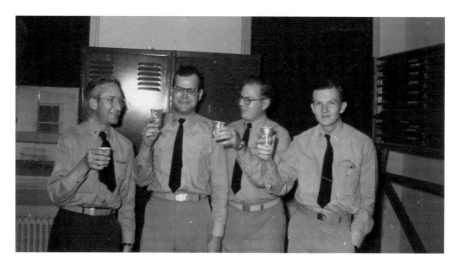

11. The navy sent me to Texas, far from any major body of water. *Left to right*: Chief of Hospital Commander Frederick Frank (the Korean War hero), Medical Officer Dr. Charles Banov, Medical Service Officer Lieutenant Tink Taylor and Medical Officer Dr. Raymond Schwartz. 1957.

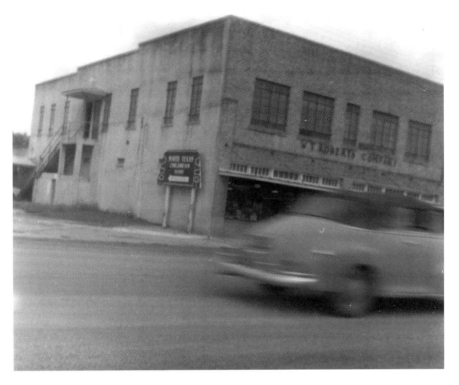

12. Pettus, Texas. My first medical office, upstairs. 1956.

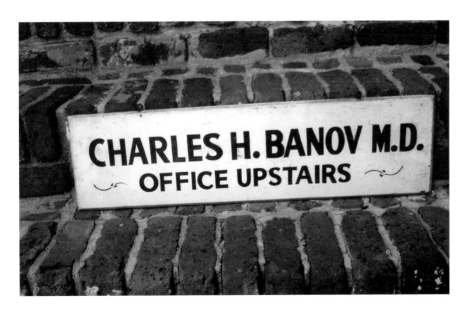

13. My sign in Pettus.

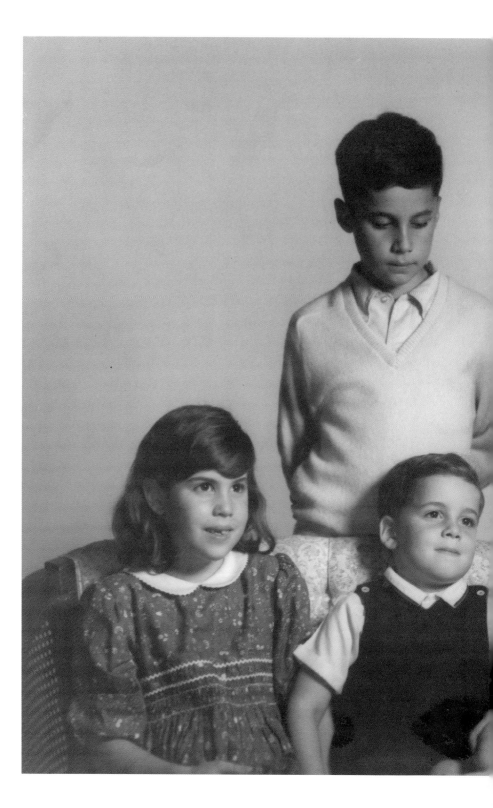

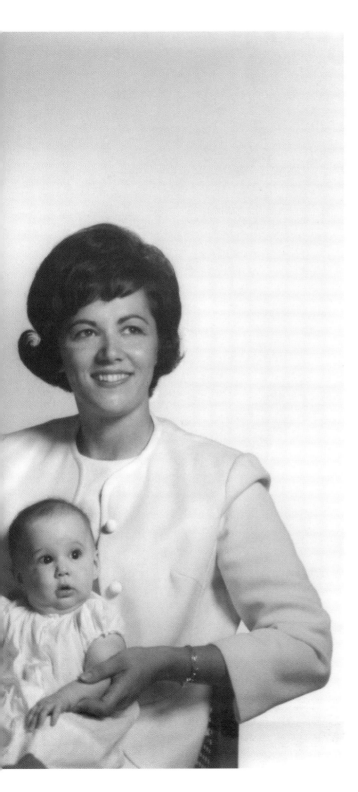

14. Nancy and our children in 1967: Mark, *standing*, and *left to right*, Lori, Michael and Pamela.

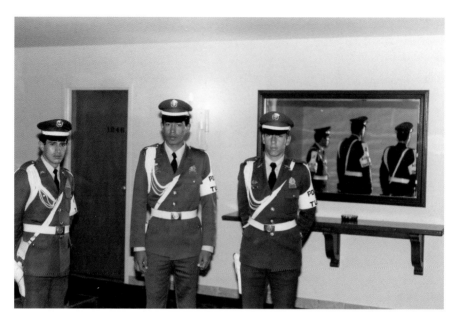

15. Overseas adventure: the three guards outside our hotel room in Bogotá, Colombia, 1986. They had been assigned to protect us from the drug lords who had threatened to kill Americans.

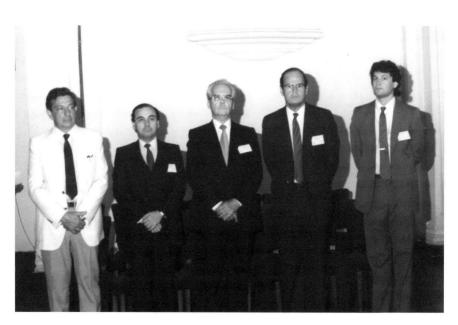

16. The grim faces may reflect concerns about the Shining Path guerillas in Lima, Peru. Not that their threats kept our son Michael, far right, from pushing the curfew—and the nerves of his father, next to him—to its limit. 1986.

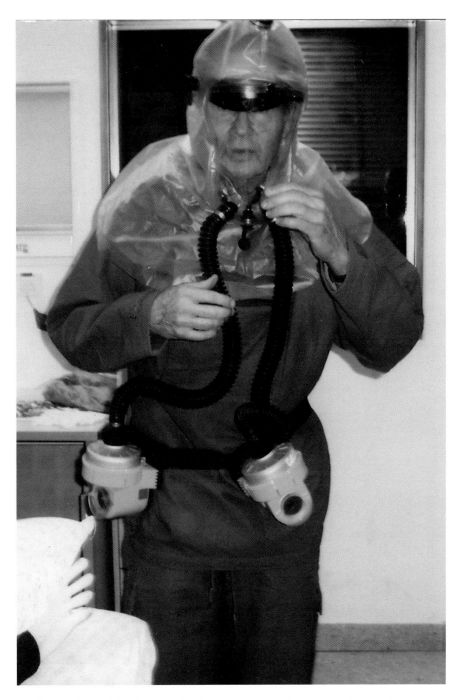

17. Bioterrorism training in Israel, 2006. I am now the oldest reserve physician in the Israeli Defense Forces, but I hope never to have to use my training.

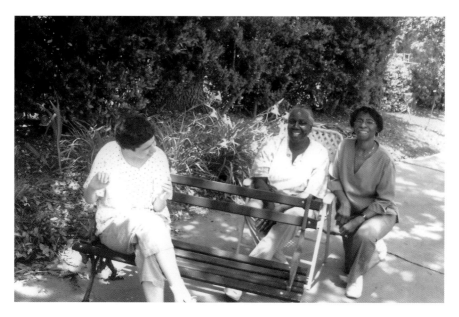

18. Three more of my heroes: our daughter Pamela and her caregivers, Ms. Helen Richards and Ms. Isabelle McBride. 2007.

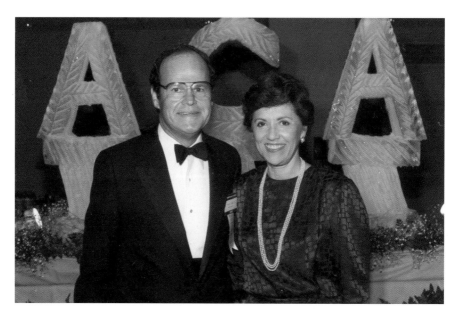

19. One of the best parts of serving as president of the American College of Allergy was being able to share the honor with Nancy. For that matter, one of the best parts of my life has been sharing it with Nancy. 1985.

"Doctor, we get good service here," she said.

"Yes, he probably gets a little special attention. I just can't help it," I replied.

"You know, he never waits when he comes into your office," she continued. "He doesn't make an appointment. He just says when he wants to come, and you immediately take him in like the president of the United States."

"You're right, but some people just become favorites in an office, and I am very touched by his thoughtfulness with the vegetables."

"Doctor, medicines are expensive, and I notice he never buys any medicine. You always give him all the medicines, no matter what they cost."

"Well, we get a few professional samples, and I like to save them for patients like your husband."

"Yeah, that old faker," said his wife. "He's been doing this with every doctor as long as I've known him. Before he goes for any medical visit, whether dentist or doctor, he buys a dollar or so worth of fruit or vegetables at the local grocery store and brings them in a bag to give to the doctor. He has never gotten a bill his entire life, never had to buy any medicines and gets the best attention in every doctor's office."

I was laughing too hard to be angry with my patient. After all, he had never said that he did not purchase those things. All he did was give me a dollar's worth of vegetables. The rest were my assumptions.

Sometimes it is what the doctor doesn't say that makes the difference, as I learned all too well.

It is an unwritten medical courtesy that when a physician interrupts another physician with a telephone call while he is seeing a patient, the receiving physician always excuses himself and takes the telephone. I was examining an asthmatic patient when the receptionist let me know that a "Dr. G." wanted to speak with me. I didn't know who Dr. G. was, but I excused myself to my patient and picked up the phone in the examining room.

The voice on the line said, "Dr. Banov, I am a veterinarian here in town, and I have a very valuable horse with heaves." Heaves is the animal model for bronchial asthma. Although I was quite flattered to be called, I wasn't sure how I could help him.

Dr. G. explained to me that he wasn't sure whether the horse had emphysema, in which case he would probably not get better and would have to be destroyed, or whether it was simply asthma, which might be reversible. He told me he had given the horse one thousand milligrams of a cortisone derivative with no response, but he didn't know what that meant.

I did know what it meant: this was a case of emphysema and could not be cured. I broke the news to the veterinarian. He asked if he should put the horse to sleep. I said I thought so. He thanked me and signed off.

When I turned back to my patient, she looked, well, scared. And why not? What she had heard went something like this: "Yes, Doctor, how can I help you?…I think you have a problem. No, the condition is not reversible…If it were my patient, I'd put him to sleep. That would be the kindest thing to do."

Needless to say, her astonishment at the half of the conversation she overheard was followed by amusement when I explained the other half.

On the other hand, it isn't always a good idea for patients to overhear both sides of a conversation. In that case, it may not be a question of misunderstanding, but of understanding all too well. When speaker telephones became available for business, I bought one right away. I thought it would be great for all concerned if doctors and patients were able to talk together in a conference call. I decided to try it out with an elderly country doctor who had referred a patient to me with liver disease. I got the doctor on the line and pushed the speaker button on my newfangled invention.

"Doctor, I have your patient, Johnny, here. You're on the speakerphone so Johnny can hear our conversation about his medical problem."

"So, that alcoholic son of a bitch showed up after all! I really didn't think he would," the physician replied, very loudly and most audibly.

"Doctor," I cut in, while trying to figure out how to turn off the speaker, "I have your patient on a speakerphone."

"I don't give a shit what kind of speaker you've got working for you. I've been carrying that bastard for years and he never paid me a dime. He also smells bad, and if he weren't my wife's cousin, I'd have shot him years ago to put him out of his miser—"

At that moment I found the "off" button. I never used the speakerphone again with a patient listening, and that referring doctor is probably still wondering why he never sees his wife's cousin in the office anymore.

It wasn't only my first patient who made me realize I needed to be sensitive to the issue of differing belief systems. But I never imagined that my patients' belief systems would influence how I practiced medicine.

One of the most lasting lessons a doctor can learn is respect for and concession to the power of faith. When Western-trained physicians speak of faith, we generally mean the Judeo-Christian concepts of prayer and religious practice. Voodoo falls outside this tradition. Believers of voodoo are thought to rely on superstition and spectacle. Until I had two patients whose very lives were threatened by the belief that they were under a voodoo spell, I really thought very little about voodoo and relegated it to the horror stories of the old Saturday afternoon movie serials.

The first patient came to me with a multitude of symptoms. Mary had lost a significant amount of weight and become increasingly physically disabled. She could barely walk. Although she was in her twenties, she looked like a sixty-year-old woman suffering from terminal cancer. When I asked her about her life to try to discover the cause of her symptoms, Mary told me that her jealous cousin, with whom she shared a boyfriend, had arranged for a voodoo priest to put a spell on her.

Not content with this explanation, I consulted one of the most respected diagnosticians, a teacher at the Medical University of South Carolina. He could find absolutely nothing wrong with her. Still, she was dying.

I could think of only one thing to do—remove the voodoo spell. I located a respected pediatric psychiatrist in the area, Dr. Ramsey Mellette, who was on the psychiatric staff of the Medical University and whose side interest was voodoo exorcism. I learned that there is an elaborate, highly prescribed way to remove a spell, involving a well-choreographed dance, drums, a snake and an animal sacrifice. I viewed film clips of such exorcisms, and Dr. Mellette added that the more established and prominent voodoo priests have a number of mysterious things they do that observers are not permitted to see.

Nothing prepared me for the actual procedure. We met at a local farm where Dr. Mellette had helped other patients suffering from voodoo spells. A chicken was sacrificed by candlelight. Its blood was spread around in a prescribed manner. Mary was rotated in different directions a number of times, and then she fell into a dream state. When she awoke, she was dramatically improved. Over the next few weeks, she regained her old self. Mary's recovery was as complete and astonishing as any I have seen.

A few years later, a similar case occurred. Sarah was an elderly woman whose sisters were angry with her for some reason. They obtained a voodoo doll and began acupuncture-like maneuvers on the doll with their knitting needles. Despite a voracious appetite and a carb-loaded diet, Sarah began losing weight. Then she developed progressive neurological changes and, finally, partial paralysis of her legs and right arm. As with Mary's case, the very best diagnosticians could find no organic basis for Sarah's ailments.

This time I was prepared. However, Dr. Mellette was completely booked, so one of his young training fellows performed the ceremony. Instead of a farm, the setting was the Medical University of South Carolina Hospital. Sarah was admitted to a general medical diagnostic floor and then transferred to a psychiatry floor. The psychiatry department agreed to allow the exorcism, more as a form of academic enrichment for the residents than in the belief that the procedure might actually be helpful.

I don't recall seeing the snake or the chicken blood at this exorcism. One of my elderly patients, who has witnessed a number of these sessions, told me that the snake and blood are always there, but are visible only to certain people. I guess I'm not one of those chosen persons who gets the orchestra seats in the voodoo world—I was raised in the belief that chicken soup cures all illnesses—but once again, within a week, Sarah, like Mary, recovered completely.

I am certain that had I not accepted the power of the voodoo faith, not to mention the assistance of professionals skilled in the practice of voodoo medicine, my patients' outcomes would have been quite the opposite.

Of course, not every phenomenon can be explained by the power of faith. Even a scientific mind must sometimes admit that there's such a thing as magic. For example, take our pregnancy chair.

One year, when our office staff was growing, we purchased a used desk chair from a nearby office furniture store. Within a month, three of our staff members, all of whom had used the chair, became pregnant unexpectedly. We chuckled at the coincidence and made little jokes about it.

Soon the patients heard about the chair and made remarks like, "Let me sit in it because I've been trying to get pregnant." Four of our patients became pregnant within the year.

As word spread—and one or two more pregnancies occurred—the jokes died away. Now we had a new problem: no one would sit in the chair. With some relief, we sold it back to the furniture store. Several months later we heard that two store employees unexpectedly became pregnant. I did not have the nerve to ask if they had used our chair.

After my first few weeks of practice, I was introduced to the little-discussed but well-recognized principle of "sluffing": a new boy on the block gives the other practitioners in the community the ideal opportunity to dump their most undesirable patients. Of course, the new doctor accepts without complaint those patients, not knowing that they are demanding, unappreciative, fail to keep their appointments, abuse the office staff, are alcoholic or depend on medications, especially pain relievers. It was an established tradition, and there was no exception. So I received Bubba, who could be charming when sober but absolutely disgusting when drunk, which was often.

Bubba was an alcoholic, pure and simple. He'd been one for years. Somehow he'd managed to hold down a job at the Charleston Naval Shipyard for many years and confine his drinking to the weekends. Alcoholics come in various colors, shapes and personalities. Some are charming and interesting, while others, like Bubba, demonstrate every disgusting characteristic, from uncontrollable body fluids and dirty clothes to horrible, abusive behavior to friends and strangers alike.

Bubba had three sisters, one of whom was Teresa Day. Miss Teresa was once married to a schizophrenic who had to be institutionalized within the first year of their marriage. She worked at a local five-and-dime, earning minimum wage and working long, exhausting hours.

Miss Teresa's one activity, besides trying to survive financially and emotionally, was taking care of Bubba when he was drinking. He would be picked up by the local police for urinating on the streets or other public excretory actions, or he would simply be found in the bushes somewhere, sleeping off a binge. The police, as well as his former doctor, knew that he could always be brought to Miss Teresa's house for care. Even though she was exhausted, she would clean up her brother, put him to bed and stay up most of the night with him so that he wouldn't choke on vomit or fall and injure himself.

Bubba's two younger sisters had married into affluent Charleston families, were well known in the social circles of our city and were, Miss Teresa told me, quite embarrassed by Bubba.

The first time I met Bubba after he was sluffed to me, he was demonstrating the worst of his affliction. This was a particularly bad episode for Bubba because he'd had a small seizure. I took him over to Miss Teresa's, but when I met her, I saw a woman who had to be one of God's angels. I just could not dump him back on her. I stayed for most of the night, mainly so Miss Teresa could get some rest. I had a chance to talk with her about her more affluent sisters. I even called each of them to tell them about her state of exhaustion and asked them to help both sister and brother.

The sisters refused to come over. Instead, each one gave me a tirade on the telephone about how bad their brother had been over the years and how they wanted nothing to do with him. If Teresa wanted to be an enabler, that was her business. They were not going to help one bit, either financially or by providing a refuge for him when he was drinking. I continued to call them, and they continued to refuse to help.

When Bubba died two years later, it turned out that he had a secret: a bank book with a very significant amount of money recorded in it. It appeared that Bubba had one element of self-control, and that was his compulsive depositing of a portion of his paycheck. No matter how down and out, he never failed to put some of his pay into that secure savings account. After many years, there was an impressive sum of money in his name. No one was more surprised than Miss Teresa.

Here was an opportunity for this unfortunate, saintly lady. She could afford to retire, tend to her flowers and find a little happiness in her life. Bubba had neglected to leave a will, but there was a note clearly giving all of his assets to Miss Teresa. The note was not signed or dated, but no one doubted its authenticity because it smelled to high heaven.

When I heard about the bank account and the note, I called the two affluent sisters and explained that here was an opportunity for their less fortunate, but faithful, sister to have some financial security. True to form, the sisters refused to give up their claims to their brother's estate.

Physicians are not supposed to become involved in their patients' financial matters, but I was so angry and upset at this injustice that I consulted my own lawyer. He became even more upset than I (and had had his own unpleasant business experiences with the family before this). He helped us speak with the probate judge, who became even more upset about the matter than my lawyer. The judge allowed a few rules to be bent, and Miss Teresa eventually got every penny of the money that Bubba left her. The sisters were disappointed, but the judge and my lawyer made it so complicated for them that it was not worth the effort to fight any longer, and they simply gave in. Miss Teresa retired and lived another ten years, tending her garden and enjoying life for the first time. Bubba's secret had a very happy ending.

Back then, even in my relatively few years of practice, I'd treated patients at both ends of the economic scale and many points in between. Still, those first years in private practice opened my eyes to yet another way needy patients were exploited, and how our health system failed them.

In those days, many insurance companies used what I consider deceptive or obstructive practices to sell policies to poorly educated, low-income patients. It worked like this: salesmen visited the homes of their customers every week to collect premiums of only a few dollars for disability and health benefits. These customers faithfully saved those few dollars every week to make the payments. The insurance policy showed benefits that were quite high, but these benefits were only paid on relatively rare diseases that the patient was unlikely to encounter. On the other hand, common conditions, such as an appendectomy, paid very little benefit, if any. The customer assumed that the policy would pay off handsomely for all medical problems; he discovered his error only when he most needed the money. Furthermore, the companies required that physicians fill out very long medical forms for the patient, sometimes on a weekly basis. This made it impractical, sometimes impossible, for the patient even to apply for payments when he needed them.

I found out about this racket when I went to see Sarah Jenkins, a sixty-eight-year-old domestic worker. She lived with her family on the third floor of a low-rent house in a once-elegant, but now rundown, area of town. There was no elevator; after my first walk up the three flights of stairs, I thought to myself that Miss Sarah, who had suffered a stroke, would not have many visitors. But I discovered that she had at least one faithful visitor every week: the insurance salesman. To my surprise, Miss Sarah handed me a multi-page medical form. This form directed that the physician complete it in full on a weekly basis, attesting to the patient's disability. The company expected that the patient simply would not get the form filled out, and the insurance company would not have to pay off its obligation. It would take as long for a physician to complete all of the questions as it would to make the house call. Of course, even after submitting the form, the insurance company never paid any additional funds.

I guess I was naïve, but I could not believe that such a situation could pass scrutiny by the regulatory agencies for insurance companies. In the 1950s and 1960s, it did.

I was young, and still capable of outrage. I purposely arranged to make a visit to Miss Sarah every week, and every week I filled out the form. After several weeks, the insurance salesman called and had the nerve to ask me if I intended to make these calls myself, or could we move the patient to a more convenient location. He knew full well that this was impossible.

I raised the issue at a Charleston County Medical Society meeting. A group of physicians and I gathered informally after that and decided to fight back for the patients against the insurance companies.

All the physicians in the group agreed to fill out as many of these forms as required, regardless of the inconvenience. This was only a first step, but what else could we do? When an attorney for one of the major hospitals pointed out that the physician's form also required the insurance salesman's signature, we had a brainstorm: we insisted that every time we filled out one of these forms the insurance agent be present to certify the validity of that signature.

Of course, after several weeks of this, a special provision to the physician's medical form was made. On long-term disabilities such as strokes, claim forms would need to be completed only every few months.

This was really going to bat for the patient, but as I have learned over the years, if we physicians don't do it, who will?

C.

Every Wednesday afternoon my father and I had lunch together. For over twenty-five years it became a tradition: he'd come to my office about an hour early and sit in my waiting room until I was ready to go. Once, walking back out to the waiting room with my last patient before lunch, I said to the patient, "You see that man there?"

I pointed to my father (who looked exactly like me, by the way—or I looked like him) and said, "You know how husbands and wives, after they live together for many years, they come to look the same? Well, you see that guy? After twenty years as my patient, don't you think he looks like me?"

My patient agreed, then went to the desk to pay his bill. As he moved to the coat closet, my receptionist motioned for me to come over and whispered, "Dr. Banov, did you insult that patient?"

"I don't think so," I said.

"Well, he wanted his records. I guess he's going to find a new doctor."

He was just putting on his coat, so I went over and asked, "Did I say something offensive?"

"No," said the patient, "but I'm taking my records because I sure as hell don't want to look like you in twenty years!"

My father and I were collaborators on another little scheme in those years, one that was dear to my heart, and no joke. Somehow the involvement of Mr. Williams in our lives struck me as the essence of Charleston.

Mr. Odell Williams, by his own admission, was always a bit slow and practically illiterate. He was a street sweeper, the kind of person who often goes completely unnoticed in a community. He was still sweeping the streets past his eightieth birthday. It certainly benefited the city for Mr. Williams to be allowed to continue working long past retirement age.

In fact, it was just about all he had in life. Mr. Williams was unmarried, lived in a single small room and took pleasure in very little besides his work. His work ethic was to be admired, and even inspired envy. I sometimes saw him at the end of the day getting on his rickety bicycle and taking his special brooms with him to prevent any coworkers from taking them. Mr. Williams's hobby was dressing up in his best clothing and sitting in the waiting room of a local hospital, simply watching the people come and go. At day's end, he got on his bicycle and went back home, returning the next day to his great capacity of street sweeper.

One day I saw Mr. Williams taking the garbage from my office and putting it out on the street. I asked him if he knew that he was not required to do this and if I could pay him for the extra service.

"But, Doctor, I must do this for you," he said indignantly. "You're my best friend."

This stunned me. I did not think I had said more than a few words to Mr. Williams, beyond, "What a nice job you do. The streets you work on probably have the cleanest gutters of any in the city." I said that half jokingly on a few occasions, when I saw him raking leaves on a rainy day and putting them into his wheeled trashcan that was almost as big as he was.

Apparently, I was the only one in about fifty years who ever commented positively on his work. This meant so much to him that he wanted to repay me by putting out my trash on a pro bono basis. When I mentioned this to my receptionist, she said, "Mr. Williams has always taken out the trash. He comes in frequently to see if you have forgotten to take any trash out. Actually, I think he welcomes any opportunity to visit with the office staff, because he gets plenty of warmth and attention that way."

That was when I cooked up this scheme with my father. We arranged for Mr. Williams to come by my father's store, Banov's Clothing Store at 595 King Street, twice a year to choose various outfits, a perk that the city certainly didn't offer.

Hanging up the Shingle

Mr. Williams, although he would not accept payment from me, seemed to find this arrangement acceptable. From then on, he went to the store in the spring and fall to pick out a pair of shoes, a shirt or two and always a large-brimmed hat. I don't know what he did with so many hats, but perhaps he counted them as part of his trophies, and wore a different one each day.

My father and I never told anyone our little secret about outfitting Mr. Williams. In fact, my father told me on many occasions that he almost had to force him to take anything more than minimal pieces of clothing. The cost of the clothing may have been a few hundred dollars a year, not more. Mr. Williams was certainly entitled to it.

When my father closed his business in 1989, we made a similar arrangement with another local merchant who also delighted in our scheme of outfitting Mr. Williams. We disguised our real intent by telling Mr. Williams that the owner of this clothing store owed me a good deal of money and wanted to pay it off in merchandise. Mr. Williams consented to do us a favor by helping us utilize these debt funds. This arrangement ended with Mr. Williams's death after a prolonged battle with a stroke. In the many months he lay in a nursing home, my staff and I were his only visitors. He was proud that his "best friends" were there to see him. He had become part of our family.

Chapter 6

Foreign Adventures

At the end of my first week in practice, I finished my only afternoon patient, looked at the four walls of my office and wondered if I'd be confined there for the next forty years. I could not have imagined that in that span of time I would visit and teach in seventy-five countries. In fact, I made so many trips abroad that I often longed for more time at home.

My wanderlust was ignited at a relatively early age. I spent the summer between college and medical school working as a merchant mariner. Ever since my aborted attempt to stow away, I'd hoped for an opportunity to go to sea. Living in a port city endowed me with a fascination for ships that exceeded any nautical skill or talent I might have had. In June of 1951, I signed on as a wiper in the engine room of an oil tanker traveling to South America. A wiper's job is easy to describe: he walks around the hot engines of the ship, wiping up excess oil. I would have preferred starting as a mess man, where I could at least wash dishes, but even after four years of college I was not qualified to do more than wipe oil from the engines.

Even if we had not been kidnapped and held for ransom, I'd have always cherished the memory of my three months with the merchant mariners. The men were almost all veterans of World War II, either as sailors or in the merchant marine itself.

There were some misfits here, people who could not adjust to unstructured civilian life and needed a programmed job and life to survive. Onboard ship, there was no need for independent decision making. Even the work itself, on a modern ship, was carefully programmed. However, not all of the crew were unable to obtain other work—many were college graduates, and quite a few had wives and children and happy home lives, despite being away for many months at a time.

During and immediately after World War II, the navy sailors deeply resented the merchant mariners, who were subject to the same dangers and discomforts as navy personnel, but received a much higher pay rate. The merchant mariners had other benefits too. For example, they ate elaborate meals not shared by the navy. Since they were not members of the military, they could bargain and complain with impunity, a luxury not shared by the sailors, though they served on the same ships, providing antiaircraft support and other military assignments. (In recent years this resentment has now re-emerged, but in reverse: now the merchant mariners want benefits provided to the military vet, such as GI college tuition and government-subsidized life insurance.) In the postwar world, though, most merchant mariners' career prospects had shrunk to little more than sequestering themselves on ships doing monotonous manual labor. They worked four-hour shifts, returned to their sparse cubicles to read girly magazines and looked forward to their one evening per month in port, when they promptly spent their entire month's pay.

My immediate superior in the engine room was Arthur Smalls, a black engineer, a graduate of the Merchant Marine Academy and my wise and kindly mentor throughout my summer on the ship.

We were docked at the port of Maracaibo, the second-largest city and second-largest port in Venezuela, along with another American tanker, when we became the target of a rebel group attempting to overthrow the government. This group commandeered any foreign ships that entered its area of unofficial authority.

I'd expected, in my naïveté, to see bandanna-wearing pirates with daggers clenched in their teeth. But these modern pirates came on board wearing white linen suits. Their behavior was almost polite, until they entered the engine room. There, a senior mate, a veteran of World War II and the celebrated and deadly Murmansk Run, informed our invaders that this was an American ship, he was an American and he would not see his American ship violated. To me, this guy was a hero nonpareil. The rebels came down the steps into the engine room, where they were met with more resistance than they expected. The cook and all of his mess men were armed with meat cleavers. The cook threw a cleaver at the rebel chief, who promptly turned and ran back up the stairs. About an hour later he reappeared, backed by fully armed, wine-inebriated rebel forces. The meat-cleaving defenders, as well as the rest of us, were marched off to a waiting bus. I assumed our next stop would be prison, followed by a firing squad.

Instead, we were taken to a place that looked to me like a motel, consisting of many individual cabins facing a courtyard. In the center of the courtyard was a sandbagged hole adorned with a large, Gatling-type machine gun. As we descended from the bus, we were given a quick salute—a machine gun blast into the air, demonstrating for us its ballistic potential.

I began to worry.

Of course, I had seen enough World War II movies to know for a certainty that the marines would come to rescue us. If my father knew of my situation, he would immediately contact our senator, the local police chief and our rabbi— each of whom, I thought, had the potential for working miracles to free us. If none of them could be reached, our employer, the American Oil Company, would surely help.

The rebels informed us that they were, in fact, in touch with our bosses on the matter of a ransom. Any decision regarding our future would depend on the company's acceptance of the rebels' terms. This made me all the more certain that the marines were on their way. But the only American military presence in the Caribbean at that moment turned out to be a nineteenth-century training schooner from Annapolis, crewed by high school students learning rope knots on their summer vacations.

We spent two terrified days and nights as prisoners, and the only thing that kept me from sinking into uncontrollable depression was the strength of Mr. Smalls, who removed a piece of wood from the adjoining door of our cells and kept up constant conversation with me, offering encouragement and confidence. If it is possible to grow up in a day or two, I did then. When any of my later foreign adventures veered into the dangerous zone, I told myself, "Well, I survived the Venezuela incident."

Some deal was made, some payment extracted from the American Oil Company and we were released. If the rebels considered this a victory, it was short-lived: the American-supported junta was firmly back in power by the next year.

That early experience did not deter me from travel, even in South America. The local political situations added a certain edge to what might have become routine medical seminars and lectures.

It wasn't always easy to assess just how dangerous a situation might be. Many years after the Venezuela incident, I traveled to Bogotá, Colombia, to teach a postgraduate course to specialists in allergy-immunology. The day before Nancy and I arrived (along with John Salvaggio, a representative of the National Institutes of Health and their wives), it happened that Carlos Lehrer, a popular figure who was head of a Colombian drug cartel, was captured in the United States. Colleagues of Mr. Lehrer in Bogotá had threatened to kill an American every day that their chief was in prison.

The American embassy informed us that we might be in great danger. We were provided with guards to ensure our safety. No one considered canceling the postgraduate course; that, we thought, would only encourage the criminals. We three American couples were placed on one floor of the hotel and all of the non-Americans were moved to other floors. Three guards with high-powered weapons were positioned outside the doors to each of our rooms. "Why three?" asked my wife. The answer was chilling: two could be bought off, but it was difficult to buy off three at a time.

At least I had the thrill of my very own personal bodyguard, an obese, elderly, avuncular gentleman who followed me everywhere I went. And I mean everywhere. He was about the last person you would expect to be a security agent, but he enabled me to experience what I imagined the president and his family must feel to have Secret Service agents around at all times. I wonder if the president has the same difficulty with urinary retention in the presence of a security agent standing behind him. I guess that's the price of leadership.

Nancy was worried, and I think she hoped that everything was being overplayed and overly dramatized. When we went to a cocktail party at the Spanish ambassador's home that evening, she expressed her concerns about safety to the wife of the U.S. ambassador to Colombia, who assured us that everything was secure and there was no danger whatsoever to Americans. I enjoyed the evening, but later on, when I happened to look out the window, I spotted the ambassador's wife leaving the party. Instead of going home in an automobile, she climbed into a small-armed vehicle escorted by U.S. Marines. We read in the newspaper a few days later that she had returned to the United States because of concerns for her safety.

During this visit, one of my Colombian colleagues told me something troubling: the Soviets were taking advantage of the political unrest in South America and America's waning support of our Latin American neighbors. They were inviting medical graduates from South America to visit the Soviet

Union for advanced training. While these graduates were given some marginal state-of-the-art training, they were also heavily indoctrinated with Soviet propaganda relative to East-West relationships. They were, in effect, buying a segment of the future intelligentsia as advocates for the Soviet cause. We, as Americans, offered nothing like that for these young, sometimes impoverished graduates.

Nancy and I decided to inform the State Department. They must not be aware of this effort, or, we thought, they would have taken some counteraction. We made an appointment with the U.S. embassy in Bogotá and were assigned to a very nice agent, who was quite concerned about what we told him. He asked if we would help with names and places, and try to collect some of the information that was being provided by the Russians to these South American physicians. We spent some of our time in Colombia doing exactly that. We were in an excellent position to learn many details through our Latin American hosts that might not be available or obvious to a formal fact-finding group. We really felt that we were of service to our government.

When we returned to the embassy, our handler told us that we needed a little basic training in intelligence gathering. We couldn't imagine how we could possibly be more discreet, so our young agent elaborated: we had faced the window when we sat in the room with the State Department interrogator assigned to the embassy. High-efficiency listening devices in another building can be trained on a speaker's lips. We should always sit with our backs to the window.

In our ventures around the city we were supposed to appear as casual pedestrians, not as American tourists. Nancy asked, "Do you think anyone really takes me for an American?"

I looked at her, with the *Herald-Tribune* in her left jacket pocket, a Walt Disney sun hat on and a tourist guide in her right pocket, and thought to myself, "Who would ever suspect that this lady is not a resident of Bogotá?"

C·Ɔ

Back in the 1960s I attended an international forum on mental health held in London. As this was my first trip to Europe, Nancy and I took the opportunity to visit France. Naturally, things did not go smoothly. First, there was some confusion with our reservations, and we found ourselves without a hotel room in Paris. A friendly receptionist at the fully booked Maurice Hotel told us about a nearby hotel, the Continental, which might have some rooms, as tourists rarely used it.

As we walked the two blocks to the hotel, I kept recalling the name Continental but could not remember where I had heard it. Suddenly it came to me that this was the hotel mentioned in the book and subsequent movie *Is Paris Burning?* During the German occupation of Paris, General Dietrich von Choltitz and his staff had used the Maurice for their headquarters. However, lower-ranking German soldiers apparently were quartered or had offices in the Continental Hotel. When the liberation of Paris took place, there was a fierce battle in the hotel. After it ended, emaciated American prisoners were found chained to a bedroom wall on the fifth floor. In other accounts of the liberation of Paris, the Continental Hotel was used by the Gestapo for interrogations.

The Continental had a room for us. That night, returning from dinner, the passenger elevator was filled, but we noticed a back elevator that seemed to open on our floor. Running that elevator was an Englishman who happened to be a World War II buff. When I told him about this hotel's particular history, he took me to the assistant manager, who led us to the basement to try to verify what was described in the book. While the fifth floor had been repaired and the moaning of the mistreated prisoners had long ago dissipated into the air of history, the basement of the Continental was unchanged from the war years of the 1940s. Nancy, the elevator operator, the assistant manager and I all went down the elevator into the past.

There were a number of mattresses stacked up, with mounds of dust blocking the exit door from the elevator. As we pushed these out of the way and opened the door, we encountered more obstructions of dust-covered items. Clearly this area had not been entered for a number of years.

Twenty-three years, in fact. No one had been in this area of the hotel since 1945. As we walked farther into the darkened area, we came upon a wall to which was attached leather straps and metal ankle restraints. The wall was peppered with bullet holes. We had uncovered the interrogation center of the Gestapo headquarters!

No one knew that the interrogation center was so intact, but as the English elevator operator told us, people were aware that this hotel had played a part in the history of the German occupation of Paris. In fact, the hotel was used two years earlier for a few scenes in the movie version of *Is Paris Burning?* Apparently they never visited the basement.

At the same time, he also told us that an overbooked tour agency had placed some of their American customers in this hotel. They were asked to use the back elevator to ease congestion on the other elevators. The actors playing the roles of the Germans, with their Nazi uniforms on, used the elevator during filming. The tourists had not been informed that there were movie scenes being filmed here. All they saw were a number of German storm troopers going up and down in the elevator. Finally, one of the guests asked our Englishman what was taking place.

"In every war," he replied, "there are some administrative people who never get the word that the war is over. These German officers have been going up and down to their office all these years. Eventually someone will tell them."

When, in the late 1980s, I received an invitation to go to Peru, I thought it would be a safe and interesting place to visit.

Nancy, who was up on current events, was not so cavalier. She had read about the Shining Path guerillas, known to be particularly vicious in the area of Machu Picchu. She bid me bon voyage and wished me luck.

However, Michael, one of our two medical student sons, agreed enthusiastically to accompany me. Upon arriving in Lima, the local police informed us that there was a curfew in all of Peru. If one were found on the street after midnight, he would be shot. If there was an accident or a problem with an automobile—if one could not get off the street by midnight—he should stop the car, open the door and lie down flat on the road, with arms and legs extended. He should explain the automotive problem to the police officer standing over him with a rifle, but there was a possibility that he would be immediately executed. That would depend on the individual police officer.

I was feeling safer already.

In South American postgraduate meetings there is always an opening ceremony. During this one, the band played the Peruvian national anthem as soldiers marched up and down the aisles of the auditorium. It was a very impressive sight. While the band played, I noticed a beautiful girl who, to my excitement, couldn't seem to take her eyes off me. When the music ended she walked straight toward me—then right past me, and up to my son, Michael. She invited him to go out with her and some friends the following Saturday night, two days away.

Saturday night came and Michael went out on his date. I had gone up to my room to sleep when I noticed it was just a few minutes before midnight and my son had not yet come in. I called the desk; they told me that this was a serious matter and that I should call the consul, which I did. A young marine at the desk told me that nothing could be done. I should just hope my son was unexpectedly delayed and that the attending troops would be merciful.

At approximately one minute before midnight I heard the rumble of military vehicles in the street. Fifteen seconds before midnight my son knocked on the door of my room and came in. He was completely calm, but by then my hands were shaking and I could barely speak, much less ask him if his date had been so wonderful that it was worth risking his life. So, like a good father, I kept my mouth shut. But I still wonder.

The next day I was asked to make grand rounds at the local medical school. Michael, who had just finished his first year of medical school, was invited along. The protocol in South American medical schools is similar to that in Europe, where the senior professor is at the head of a long line of junior professors, instructors, residents, interns and, finally, medical students, in decreasing proximity to the patient.

The senior professor was always very happy to have guests from other countries make rounds with him, for one reason— a disease called verruga peruana, transmitted by a sand fly unique to a thirty-mile radius of Lima, Peru, and no other place in the world, except for the rare outbreak in other South American countries. The lesions on the leg are well demarked and very specific for this disease. The senior professor enjoyed quizzing all visiting medical dignitaries to see if they had any hint of what this locally common condition was. So he was extremely disappointed when Michael's turn came at the bedside of a sufferer of this unique type of bartonella. Michael was able to diagnose him immediately. The reason he knew the answer was that freshman medical students study obscure things they will never need. Or not unless they happen to be seeing a patient in Lima, Peru, and making rounds with a senior professor.

At the South American postgraduate meetings, I could always count on a national anthem, as well as something more exciting. One memorable opening ceremony took place before a course in Buenos Aires, Argentina. While the Argentine national anthem was being sung, the director of the course came over to me and whispered in my ear, "Well, Doctor, are you ready for your talk?"

I said that I was, but added that this was only Thursday night. My talk was Saturday morning.

"Not your scientific lecture. I meant your social lecture."

I asked him what in the world my social lecture was.

He pointed to the television cameras around the auditorium and said, "Why, you are the main speaker tonight. Right after the opening ceremony."

After a short silence, I asked what my subject was.

"Don't you remember?" he asked. "When I contacted you I asked you to speak about the improvement or lack of improvement of professional relationships between North and South American physicians."

Nancy thought this was hilarious. I didn't. Should I confess that I had never received this notification, or should I try to bluff my way through? Nancy wasn't helping with the decision. "Let's see how you get out of this one!" she said.

At the end of the national anthem, I moved to the podium and began my talk. Nancy condescended to feed me questions and statements, and we somehow produced a completely extemporaneous, forty-five-minute plenary lecture, which was well received. The local media wrote glowing descriptions of the desire of Americans to cooperate with the new North-South spirit.

In addition to their opening ceremonies, the South American medical professional community has other customary activities that might be hard to believe to one who hasn't been there. These folks know how to have a good time. They have very serious medical meetings during the day, but at night they have plenty of energy for carnival-like activities that include periods of wild, frenzied dancing.

There is no warning when the dancing will begin or end. It is up to the orchestra. One could be in the midst of a serious award presentation, and then receive a signal from the bandleader indicating that at the end of a presentation the dancing will begin.

The scientific lectures are a bit more organized, although they follow the principle of *más o menos*, which in Spanish means "more or less." If one is to present a formal lecture, it may be listed in the program for five o'clock but not begin until nine o'clock, with some dancing and perhaps an unscheduled light meal in between. The main meal may not begin until midnight. If the host is to pick you up at the hotel at eight o'clock, he may arrive one to two hours later. After a while, a seasoned medical lecturer, which I thought myself to be, may decide to buck the system and arrive a mere hour late, only to find that the host arrived at exactly the right time, and the lecture hall is filled with a punctual (just that once), impatient audience.

At these meetings one always receives an elaborate plaque or diploma. Some of them are very large and beautifully designed. I collected a number of these awards over the years, and Nancy decided it would be an effective decorating scheme to hang them in one examining room. We put a good deal of thought into the appropriate arrangement on the wall. But the first patient who came into the examining room looked at the wall and said, "You seem like a good doctor. Why did you have to go to South America to study medicine?"

We took down the awards.

In 1976 I thought that any fears of kidnapping were well in my past, or at least beyond the borders of my own country. But I was wrong.

It happened one summer afternoon. I was busy in my office seeing patients when my receptionist buzzed me to say that my wife was on the phone. I knew it must be urgent because Nancy would never normally call me during office hours. Nevertheless, I was shocked at her opening statement: "Charles, they've got Lori!"

She had received a telephone call. The voice at the other end said calmly, "Listen carefully. We have your daughter. This is not a crank call."

He then recited all of our teenage daughter's clothing sizes, from her blouse to her underwear. He obviously had Lori. At that moment, my son picked up the extension and asked, "Who is this?" The caller hung up.

My wife sat there in horror. It so happened that a terrible kidnapping, resulting in the deaths of two teenagers, had occurred at nearby Folly Beach some time earlier.

At that time, Lori was receiving guitar lessons from a male instructor in an area close to where that crime had occurred. Although the murderer had been caught, the recollection of the details of the crime, in which the two children were slowly hanged, was fresh in our minds. Although this instructor was known to some of the teenagers and was recommended by our daughter's friends, we did not know his address. We did know the telephone number, but I was afraid that if he were indeed the kidnapper and our daughter's life was truly in danger, then a call from the police or from us, unless it was very carefully handled, could result in a tragedy.

For some reason, I was calmer and more in control of my emotions than I would have expected. Perhaps my training as a physician in emergencies, or maybe the fact that I watched enough TV and heard enough horror stories, enabled me to know that there were steps to be taken. I simply did not want an inexperienced officer sending a group of siren-wailing police cars in the direction of our jeopardized daughter.

I called the chief of police, who I knew, but he was out of town. One of my boyhood friends and current patients was an FBI agent in town, and I was able to get in touch with him immediately. He told me that according to FBI protocol at that time, they could not enter the case for forty-eight hours, unless there was some proof that our daughter had been taken out of the state.

This was obviously a local matter. After we called the police, a cordial but obviously inexperienced officer arrived at our home. I instructed him to contact his supervisors to see if a kidnap crisis team could be quickly organized, or if we could get some advice from experts on how to proceed.

By then I'd learned that our neighbor's daughter was to have a lesson from the same instructor within the next hour. She was preparing to drive out there. I got into my car and followed her out to the instructor's house.

At some point during the thirty to forty minutes in which all of this occurred, I realized that if the police could not become organized and demonstrate that they had an appropriate team to handle the matter, I would have to do something myself. My office manager reminded me much later that she knew it was serious because I stopped by the office to pick up a gun, and she knew I had the determination to use it if necessary.

Following my neighbor's child to a possible kidnap scene was not the nicest thing I could have done to a neighbor and friend, but I was desperate. There was no way I could tell the police where she was located because I did not know. It took less than thirty minutes to reach the guitar instructor's home, but during that drive, I found out a good deal about myself and my ability, if necessary, to kill another human being. If my daughter had been harmed, I decided I could and would shoot the individual responsible on the spot. I made this decision calmly and with thought of all the repercussions, but I would not allow anyone who had harmed my child to walk away unscathed.

Meanwhile, the police simply called the phone number. My daughter was there, unharmed. The guitar instructor knew nothing about a kidnapping. But had he been the perpetrator, and had a crime been committed, that telephone call could have been disastrous.

I arrived before the police. I got out of the car and walked toward the house. As I did so, the door opened and out ran the instructor with his hands in the air, and Lori, running a bit faster—just as the police had instructed them to do.

All I could see was my daughter running and a man with his hands in the air. I yelled for Lori to drop to the ground (which, she recently reminded me, she did not do). With the gun held on him, I told her instructor to remain exactly where he was—any movement would be his last. Within a few minutes, the police arrived, sirens blaring. They quickly verified that no crime had been committed. Only then did I lower the gun.

The kidnap story was a gigantic hoax. It happened to a number of people in a three-week period. A police task force was formed and the victims were brought together. They all told the same story: the day before the kidnap phone call, a call was made to those homes that had domestic help. The caller said he was from the Sears-Roebuck Company, and that someone wished to give the teenager in the home a gift of some clothing. Would the housekeeper check the closet and give him the sizes of the various garments that would be assembled as a gift?

Since this was to be a surprise, the housekeeper was cautioned not to tell anyone about it, or the surprise would be ruined. Seven other people also were taken in by the ruse. Ours was complicated by the fact that our daughter was taking lessons in the area where a murder had recently occurred and was out of the home when the call came. In all of the other calls, it became apparent after a short period that this was a hoax, but ours was just the wrong circumstance at the wrong time.

The perpetrator was indicted, charged and punished for his antics. All was well—except that I found that I had the potential to take a life. This left a disturbing mark on me that I would never forget.

I recently asked Lori, now the mother of four children, what she remembered about the ordeal and why she did not comply with my command to drop to the ground. I'd never really discussed the incident with her since it happened, wary of initiating recall of a suppressed memory—the psychiatric stuff we were taught in medical school. But her answer revealed the mind of a teenager at work: "Dad, I remember it all very well. It was the most embarrassing moment of my life!"

So much for being a hero to my children.

Chapter 7

A Community
of Special People

If we are lucky in life, we get to know extraordinary individuals who, for one reason or another, simply stand out from the crowd. They may not be famous or financially successful, but we recognize them for sterling qualities that enrich their acquaintances and their world. I've known a lot of special people in my life. I can't help it if a few of them are my relatives.

Our customs in the South are well entrenched. The first thing one learns in early childhood is to be respectful of one's elders, and this means not calling them by their first names unless we are within a year or two of their ages. "Cousin" is what we Southerners call those people who mean the most to us. The term "cousin" can mean anyone from a first to a fourth cousin, but also means a relative who is too adult to have his or her first name used.

I could never allow myself to call Dr. Leon Banov Sr. by his first name, even when I was in my fifties and he was still a practicing physician. I held him in such esteem that even though our families were close and I saw him often, I could not be on a first-name basis with him. Calling him "Dr. Banov" seemed too formal, even at professional events, so I compromised on the still-respectful title of "Cousin Leon."

Cousin Leon started out as a practicing pharmacist in a local drugstore in Charleston. Then he went to medical school and became a physician interested in public health. As a matter of fact, he was one of the first trained public health officers in the United States. Through his efforts, in 1919 Charleston became the first city in the world to enact an ordinance requiring milk to be pasteurized before it was sold. Before the ordinance, dairies pasteurized milk only for calves. According to Cousin Leon's memoirs, the pedigreed calves were so valuable that dairies could not afford the risk of giving them raw milk. Cousin Leon argued for the ordinance by asking city hall if "human babies are not just as valuable as calves." The rest of the country and most of the world followed suit, with the result that millions of people were spared disease.

Cousin Leon was the director of the Charleston County Health Department from 1936 to 1962, but had been associated with the preventive medicine programs of our city for more than fifty-seven years. He turned down many opportunities, such as being director of public health for the state and city of New York. He preferred to be a public health officer, helping with home deliveries and immunizations and trying to solve the tremendous maternal and infant mortality problems in the South. He retired as the health officer for Charleston County when he was in his seventies.

Feeling that he still had many years of wisdom to share, he undertook a full residency in psychiatry. After completing the residency, he practiced psychiatry and at the same time qualified as a hematologist. In his eighties, while practicing hematology (and a little psychiatry on the side), he was killed in an automobile accident on his way to a medical meeting. At his memorial service I eulogized Cousin Leon by relating a fantasy:

> Somewhere in Heaven, all the great medical scientists of history were present in their own fraternity, and among such people as Louis Pasteur, Oliver Wendell Holmes Sr. and the sixteenth-century surgeon Ambrose Paré sat Cousin Leon. I do not know what they discussed up there in Heaven, but this I know: if Cousin Leon were

up there, every angel in Heaven had had his tetanus and smallpox immunizations.

Dr. Leon Banov was my role model and my mentor. At the end of my first day of medical school, I came home to find him sitting on the porch, waiting for me. He held an old, worn box. Inside it was a stethoscope, also worn. I didn't need to ask whose stethoscope it was. Cousin Leon told me that he was delivering this to me from my grandfather, who would have liked nothing better than to give this to me himself. That was my grandfather, Sam Banov—the immigrant, merchant and unofficial doctor, who never spent a day in medical school but whose big medical book was consulted to heal indigent newcomers to America. Cousin Leon understood how much it would have meant to my grandfather to see me become a doctor.

Years passed. Cousin Leon's son, Dr. Leon Banov Jr., who was closer to my age, became a proctologist, and I became an allergist. We had offices on the same street. We were affiliated with the same hospital. Naturally, we became known as "Heads and Tails." Our similar names and opposite specialties made life miserable for our receptionists and frustrated the hospital staff. Patients would be asked to make appointments with a Dr. Banov for itches, congestion or stuffiness. Their symptoms, however they described them, seemed to indicate either one of us. Patients with painful rear ends were often sent to me for testing for ragweed and cat allergy. Then, after yet another disappointed patient left the office in search of the correct Dr. Banov, I could hear the office staff whisper, "Wrong end."

There are certain patients in a physician's practice who are simply special. Admittedly, that special patient might be a prominent businessperson, a famous community leader or even the physician's personal accountant. My office is no exception. I like to think our special patients gained that status not because of their fame or notoriety, but because of something in their past relationship with the office that is unique and precious.

I first met Dorothy in 1961, when I'd been in practice for only two weeks. My wide-open schedule and blank appointment book allowed me the opportunity to volunteer at a local center for persons with mental retardation, the Coastal Center for the Developmentally Disabled. As I made my rounds on a very dark, gloomy ward that reeked of urine, I saw a three-year-old child lying on a rug in a fetal position. Her roommates were twenty-four of the most deformed, unattractive and difficult-to-treat children. Some had malformed heads; some were afflicted with multiple deformities, such as missing fingers and ears; some were unable to walk or develop in any way. These children were destined to spend their short lives in this institution. Dorothy looked different from the others. I discovered that she was suffering from severe asthma due to reflux of swallowed secretions, which severely irritated her lungs. While she had been kept clean and free of bedsores, little attention was given to her asthma. I brought the child to the infirmary, and her asthma was treated appropriately, as was the reflux.

Her medical condition improved dramatically, and so did her mental state. It was clear that she should not be on that ward, nor should she have been sentenced to spend her life with those children. Dorothy was only minimally retarded. Her true mental status was masked by her medical problems, and those may have been worsened by the institutional life she had lived so far.

Those were the days before Medicaid, Medicare or the various government subsidies that are now available for children with disabilities. My office staff and I enthusiastically took on this child as a special project. Dorothy was soon released from the institution and placed in a special school, where she quickly developed, both physically and intellectually. She graduated from high school, went to trade school to become a nurse's aide and met her future husband. She lives a beautiful, productive and enjoyable life. Her asthma treatment needs follow-up and adjustment, which means she has periodic checkups with me. She once said that when she comes in for an appointment she is treated like a queen. Her family is jealous, she tells us, because when she walks into my office everyone stands up.

Part of the orientation of all new personnel in my practice for the past thirty-eight years is a recitation of the story of Dorothy. I've noticed a tear or two in the eyes of many staff members when they tell it. Her ability to enjoy her life for these years has been one of the greatest pleasures in my practice of medicine.

I know there are many people in the world like Dorothy. They are the fuel that powers my professional life.

The practice of medicine is a continuous learning experience, and so is life. Sometimes we're given lemons and sometimes lemonade. I always had a pitcher full of the latter until 1968. Then life took a sudden turn.

After seven years of practice, I thought I was quite experienced in unusual situations and felt confident that I could handle whatever came along, either professionally or personally. I had three normal children and took for granted their ability to learn language, walk and respond to expressions of love and attention. I accepted their hugs when I came home, their enjoyment of bedtime stories and their growing understanding of a "yes" or a "no" from their parents. I used to receive the request for another glass of water or another bedtime story in order to delay sleep with the usual irritation of a tired parent. It never occurred to me, when I'd look forward to my children's toilet training between two and three years of age, that some children entered adulthood without becoming toilet trained, or could never distinguish between acceptable and unacceptable behavior. Little did I realize that the hug of a normal child wishing to delay sleep was so precious that it could never be fully cherished.

Our fourth child, Pamela Rae Banov, was born on the Fourth of July, 1966, a beautiful and apparently normal child. We took for granted the fact that she had all of her fingers and toes, two ears and a little hair on her head. We expected the normal developmental stages: grasping our fingers, crying appropriately and learning to move her head, arms and legs in coordination. I never even noticed these things as they occurred. Parents-to-be often worry before the first child is born, but after two or three a certain complacency sets in. Of course, everything will be fine.

Sometime around Pamela's eighth month, strange things began to occur with her. She appeared to have hearing loss, because she would not respond to our "yes" and "no" commands. As she grew older, we noticed that when she turned on the water faucet and we said "no," she would simply turn on the other faucet. There was no eye contact. No speech, except for horrible screams at night, as if she were in pain. I learned the difference between normal crying and inappropriate crying. She would not sleep and appeared to remain upright in bed all night long, or she would suddenly get out of bed and not respond to commands. Nor did she respond to touching, feeling or the warmth offered from a parent to a child.

She was frightening.

About that time, there appeared, both in lay literature and in medical journals, a description of a little-understood condition known as autism. Autistic children were often labeled schizophrenic and were tucked away in institutions and forgotten. With the advent of modern psychiatry and sophisticated pediatric neurology it became apparent that there were many more autistic children than the scientific world had realized.

With great difficulty, we took Pamela to New York to see a child psychiatrist, a woman said to be one of the world's greatest authorities on autism and child psychoses. She was not able to see us for months, though her assistant, a psychologist, could see us sooner. But all the psychologist could tell us was that Pamela was indeed autistic, and nothing could be done.

We left that session devastated.

Nancy and I had accepted the fact that our child had a major developmental disability, but we thought that something could be done—maybe by us, at least by someone. To have an authority on the matter exclaim, "I don't know what to do, and no one does," was a cruel blow. I have remembered that feeling ever since, and considered it in my medical practice. There is always something that can be done for every condition, no matter how hopeless—if not to cure, then to comfort. In the words of Sir William Osler, "To heal sometimes, but to comfort always." I see some mighty sick people in my practice, but I always give them hope—not untruths or false hopes, but something to do. Never do I say that I don't know what to do.

Back then, the ignorance about this developmental disability was appalling. In fact, a prevailing school of thought was that autism was caused by some unconscious rejection of the child by the parents. One recommended therapy, according to these experts, was a "parentectomy"—take your child to an institution and leave her without family contact for many years. Parents were not even allowed to visit and only received periodic reports. All this was considered to be in the best interest of the child. We know now that this is the wrong approach.

We tried to find facilities for treatment, first here in South Carolina and then elsewhere in the United States. Pamela was becoming increasingly difficult to manage at home. We learned that other people—many others, some quite prominent—had autistic children. We weren't alone.

Since no programs existed in our state, Nancy made up her mind that she would create them. And that's what she did.

A Community of Special People

We approached our U.S. senator, Fritz Hollings, for assistance in submitting a bill for research and programs to the Congress. Senator Hollings arranged for us to testify before a Senate committee. My testimony and Nancy's were supported by actors Lloyd Nolan and Tony Curtis, who had family members with similar difficulties.

On March 21, 1973, the *New York Times* reported:

> *Speaking calmly of their own families, actors Tony Curtis and Lloyd Nolan appeared before the Senate Subcommittee on the Handicapped to lend their support to legislation to increase federal aid for the nation's 7 million handicapped children. Mr. Curtis told of a brother in a mental institution since childhood and of two daughters who had learning difficulties. Mr. Nolan spoke of a son who suffered from autism and died four years prior at the age of 26.*

The result was that autism was listed under the Developmental Disabilities Act, along with mental retardation, epilepsy and cerebral palsy, to provide for programs to assist these children and their families.

When Pamela was diagnosed, South Carolina had absolutely no facilities for diagnosis and treatment of autism. Today the state has a multimillion-dollar budget to serve the growing autistic population.

Years later, our daughter received the appropriate diagnosis of Rett syndrome, which has subsequently been found to have a nonhereditary, genetic origin. The actual gene has been identified. Although there has been no success yet in treating this condition, it can now be identified before birth.

This story is not only about one child and one condition, but about a group of people who are certainly special—the whole family of a special needs child. I had the opportunity to meet and become a part of the fraternity of people with special children. I am convinced that whatever deity exists in this world assigns these children to certain families for a reason. There is a love and bond between special-needs children and their parents that is hard to imagine. It is easy to love a normal child, even one who has difficulty with school or social situations, or with drugs or crime. But many special-needs children offer nothing in return—no eye contact, no response to a kiss. They withdraw when touched. The parents of these special children find love in a brief moment of eye contact, a touch of the finger or a small smile that only the parent is privileged to see.

That is true love.

These parents are often tired, and are always under emotional strain. There are occasional broken marriages as a result, although many marriages, such as ours, are strengthened by this challenge. Often the parents are burdened with extra work in order to pay for their child's care. Yet the parents are probably the world's most effective advocates for their child's cause. Their power and ability to make themselves heard is phenomenal.

When things don't go right in business, medicine or sports, I've heard people ask, "Why me?" I rarely hear the parent of a special-needs child ask, "Why me?" In fact, many parents, when they first receive their child's diagnosis, feel, as I did, "If not us, then who?" Parents are too busy caring for their child to have time for self-pity. Many of them work for the entire community by fighting the rampant abuse suffered by mentally handicapped persons living in group homes or in inadequately and improperly staffed facilities. People like Nancy are devoting their lives to making legislators aware of the deficiencies of laws protecting handicapped persons, many of whom cannot speak for themselves, whose families must accept the appearance of fresh bruises on their institutionalized loved ones as the result of "accidental falls," when they know better. But that's another story to be told, one that will be told by their families.

A Community of Special People

My seatmate on an airplane trip some years ago was a physician returning from Vietnam to make some financial arrangements for his ninety-four-year-old mother, who lived in a nursing home. This physician told me that he felt guilty about spending large amounts of money on his mother while young children were dying in Vietnam for lack of basic necessities. He knew he could have saved more lives had he taken that money and given it to Vietnamese orphanages. He agonized over his situation for some time until he realized, more clearly than before, that every life is precious. One cannot decide which life is more appropriate to be saved.

Two special people in our daughter Pamela's life are Mrs. Isabelle McBride and Ms. Helen Richards. They are aides who came to us many years ago to help with our daughter and have become probably the world's most skilled therapists and caretakers of an individual with Rett syndrome. These two delightful people have worked together, but rarely at the same time, for over thirty years. They are brilliant, dedicated, highly skilled professionals who have devoted their entire life's work to a perpetual child who will never be able to thank them. They have the ability to communicate, through a secret language known only to them and to God, with a severely neurologically damaged individual, and have given her a quality of life that could never have been achieved otherwise. They derive satisfaction from the fact that they can get our child, at forty-one, to go into a swimming pool or for a long walk, and to say a few words. There is a special love between Pamela and these two very important people in her life. Mrs. McBride and Ms. Richards rate, in my book, with all of the famous or near-famous people I have ever known.

Our three other children are another group of special people. Like other siblings of special needs children or adults, they have been tested under the fire of trying to extract love from a non-verbal and non-responsive sister.

Since early childhood they heard the whispers of cruel immaturity from their friends: "What's wrong with your sister?" They learned not to be quite so embarrassed when a new schoolmate came to our home and heard a blood-curdling scream. Sometimes we expect those things when we visit aged relatives in nursing homes, but to a teenager with a teenager's fragile ego, a sibling in the home with mental retardation is a bit of a resented strain.

Yet I find that most of the normal siblings of these retarded persons are protective of their "little brothers" or "little sisters," who will remain as such all their lives. Our other three children are themselves more patient, considerate and appreciative of their own children as a result of their living with a special needs sibling. Even our unmarried physician son Mark has a natural warmth and ability to communicate with his young patients that I feel certain was learned in our home from a child who cannot talk, but who teaches love and understanding simply by being here.

Chapter 8

Wheezes, Sneezing and Itches

Gradually, as my specialty became more established, my practice shifted from general internal medicine to focus exclusively on allergy.

Until the mid-1960s, there was considerable difference in the quality of care provided by the internist (the specialist in internal medicine) and the family practitioner. It was customary for the family doctor to have only a year of a rotating internship, after which he was expected to take care of children from birth to adulthood, and even to perform surgical procedures such as tonsillectomies and appendectomies. The internist had an additional three years of formal training, excluding surgery, obstetrics and pediatrics. He or she treated everything from a viral sore throat to a heart attack. The internist was the consultant called in by the general practitioner to solve a difficult diagnostic puzzle. Eventually, as subspecialization grew, the general internist became the family doctor. The subspecialist became the consultant.

When subspecialization became the standard, I reluctantly gave up my internal medicine practice and focused on allergy and immunology. I loved the detective work of my specialty, though I sometimes missed the remarkable array of medical problems, curious patients, unique situations, excitement and triumphs that came to me as an internist.

Early in my practice, an attractive young woman, a recent college graduate who was about to be married in a few weeks, came to see me. She had mentioned to previous physicians in years past her total amenorrhea—lack of a menstrual cycle— but they had chosen not to investigate its possible causes. Finally, almost on the eve of her wedding, her gynecologist referred her for endocrinological evaluation.

Up until the most recent years, most diagnostic puzzles were referred to the internist. Subspecialists such as endocrinologists remained in their ivory towers at the university hospitals, seeing private patients only for a few hours each week. So it was logical that I would see many cases of endocrine problems in my internal medicine diagnostic practice.

I ordered a test—chromosomal analysis, through a scraping of skin cells from the inside of the cheek—as an appropriate tool to help diagnose the patient's problem. Perhaps it would have been better had I not done so. The test revealed that our young bride-to-be was, in fact, male.

What should we do? After twenty-three years of female life, should we tell her that she was really a man? How would her friends and family feel? How would her fiancé react? Late one afternoon I assembled the physicians involved in the case in my office. We agreed that ethics and legality be damned, we would find some way to keep this tremendous revelation from her. The patient psychologically was a female and should be kept a female.

Of course, there would be repercussions from this decision. Obviously, the marriage would be infertile; we didn't tell her. She would need estrogen supplements, and some anatomical rearrangements—a surgical procedure would create a functioning vagina. But how could we explain the surgery and still keep the secret?

We asked her father to come in for a conference. A biochemist by profession, he understood the biological situation and appeared to be extremely sympathetic and eager to cooperate. But he was also a very religious man and after leaving my office he decided to get a second opinion from his priest. The priest's opinion was emphatic and uncompromising: the patient must be returned to her original sex.

Her father could not accept that point of view, and appealed to higher authorities in the church. He always got the same answer. Ultimately, we were forced to tell the young lady the truth about herself. Three days later, I assisted in detoxifying her from a drug overdose requiring hospitalization and a good deal of prayer.

The marriage was postponed and the surgery was performed. After a few months, the couple broke their engagement and severed their relationship. Some twenty years later, I heard that my patient had died in an automobile accident on her way to a health food festival. She never married, and I know nothing about her relationships with men or women, but I suspect that they were difficult to sustain.

Physicians often wrestle with the problem of how much information to share with a patient. What about some of the terrible newborn diseases, which invariably produce suffering followed by premature death? Certainly, techniques exist to anticipate these problems and to give the mother-to-be some choice about whether to chance a completed pregnancy. Nevertheless, if that window of opportunity is missed, and the child is born with a disease, how much information should we give the parents? It is so difficult to decide, and it takes tremendous psychological insight into the patient to know how to do this in a kind way. Still, this is the responsibility of a caring physician and is not a task that can be relegated to anyone else. The purpose of the art of medicine should be to help patients enjoy the maximum quality of life.

For example, the daughter of an aristocratic, eighty-eight-year-old Charleston lady called me one day, saying, "Mother has flipped her lid!" The daughter found her completely naked, jumping up and down on her bed, cursing to beat the band.

I came over to see for myself. A diabetic, the patient had taken too much insulin that morning, dropping her blood sugar to a dangerous level. The imbalance temporarily affected her brain, and she lost all of her inhibitions. This reserved and appearance-conscious dowager desperately wanted to do something bad. With her background, profanity seemed to be the worst thing she could think of. Even so, she apparently had learned only two curse words in her long, sheltered life. So there she was, buck naked, jumping on the bed, screaming, "Hell, damnit, damnit, hell, damnit, hell, hell, damnit…"

A glass of orange juice with a teaspoon of sugar in it produced a dramatic recovery and some blessed forgetfulness on the lady's part. Neither the family nor I had the heart to tell her how she had acted when her brain received an insufficient amount of sugar.

There's one aspect of the medical profession that I think does not exist in quite the same way in any other: you're always a doctor, wherever you go. It's difficult, if not impossible, to be completely "off duty" in any situation. While a physician cannot experience all of the possible situations that can occur in medicine, he has been trained with enough basic information to extemporize and adjust to any situation. Sometimes this requires a mixture of luck, experience, ingenuity and even a bit of politics.

Many years ago, I boarded an airplane for a lengthy flight from Israel to the United States. A fellow passenger, while walking onto the plane, was accidentally struck in the eye by another passenger. His injury didn't seem very serious until the flight was well underway and we were out of reach of land. The man's eye became quite swollen, and he was in extreme pain. The flight attendant placed cold compresses on the eye, but after another hour or two in flight his condition worsened.

A call was sent out for any doctor on board. A musician with a PhD, a piano tuner and a veterinarian all raised their hands. It looked as if I was the only medical professional in the group, so I volunteered my services.

I knew enough to know that I didn't know enough about eye injuries to tell if this man was in an emergency situation. But I didn't want to risk making the wrong decision and causing him to lose the eye. I had heard about a service where specialists were on call to give advice in an emergency to people in remote places, far from medical care. The middle of the ocean ought to qualify as remote, I thought.

Now things were getting interesting. I was invited up to the inner sanctum of the cockpit to use the radio. With the navigator's help, I called a number of governmental agencies without results. Finally, I reached my own family ophthalmologist, who was quite surprised to hear from me in the middle of the Atlantic Ocean. He confirmed that I truly had an emergency, but that the only help I could give the patient was pain relief. Further treatment would have to wait until he could get to a hospital.

The patient had asked to be taken off the plane in Iceland. I discussed with the pilot whether we should land in Iceland, with great inconvenience to all the travelers and great expense to the airline. I couldn't tell if it was medically necessary.

The pilot said that he was not a doctor, but he would use the Israeli army's medical questionnaire to evaluate the man. I'd never heard of such a thing.

"It's an effective diagnostic tool," he said. "I'll show you how it works." We went over to the patient, and the pilot introduced himself.

"If you are in such great pain, sir, we'll land the plane in Iceland," said the pilot.

"Yes, I can't stand it much longer," replied the patient.

"All right," continued the pilot. "Of course you will be quarantined for three weeks, won't be able to conduct business during that time and will most likely remain isolated in the hospital for another few weeks for insurance purposes. Then you will be allowed to go home." He looked at the patient. "Now, how bad is your pain?"

The man said it was that bad.

"We'll land in Iceland. This man is really sick," said the pilot.

The pilot's ability to evaluate pain, with the help of his army questionnaire, clearly was greater than mine. The man's eye was saved because of the medical attention he received in Iceland.

There are plenty of instances in which I try to avoid letting people know that I'm a physician. Nancy and I once took a three-day cruise to the Caribbean after a particularly exhausting few months in my practice. On these ships, passengers took their meals at the same table with the same people for the entire cruise. Were these folks to know that I was a physician, I feared that all we would talk about were their medical problems or experiences. I really needed a rest; I wanted to be away from medicine completely for a few days.

Nancy and I decided to tell our table companions that I was a naval engineer. If anyone asked me specific questions, I planned to say that my work was top secret and I could not discuss any of it. That was a delightful decision, and not only because it made me feel like a secret agent. For the first time in many years, there was no talk whatsoever of medicine. If the subject did come up, I was simply a bystander to the conversation.

I kept up my charade until the final night when, at the captain's party, a seventy-four-year-old man, on the cruise for his third honeymoon, stood up, grabbed his chest in a classic sign of coronary distress and said, "Boy, do I have a stomachache!" It was perfectly clear to me that he was having a heart attack. I went with the man to a nearby lounge, where he lay down on a couch to wait for the arrival of the ship's doctor, a retired obstetrician-gynecologist whose post-retirement years were spent treating benign cases of seasickness and sunburns. I told the doctor that I was a physician and that I was turning the patient over to him for care. The doctor thanked me and I left the room.

The next morning, I saw the doctor at breakfast and asked him what had happened to our patient. "What is the protocol for a situation like this?" I asked. "Is the patient airlifted off the ship, or is there an intensive-care facility onboard to monitor him?

"What are you talking about?" replied the doctor, giving me a puzzled look.

"What did the electrocardiogram show?" I asked.

"Man, that machine is heavy, and it's on the other side of the ship," he said. "I'm not about to lug that thing all the way over here."

I was amazed. I was certain that the man had had a heart attack and had been in real trouble, but the doctor just pointed across the room. "There's the fellow, over there."

I looked over and saw my dinner companion, methodically consuming a large platter of pancakes with syrup. In other words, eating like a teenager who'd never heard the words "myocardial infarction."

I would've bet my reputation that this man had had a heart attack. Ten years from now, I thought to myself, someone will take an electrocardiogram of him and ask if he had a heart attack in the past. The man will be surprised at the question and answer, "No, not at all. As far as I know, I have never had any problems with my heart."

On the other hand, had the man been closer to competent medical care, he would have spent his third honeymoon in an intensive-care unit with bells ringing and tubes running in and out. Maybe sometimes it is better not to know too much.

Even a planeload of experts is sometimes no match for a determined layperson. One year our state medical society was beginning a European tour when one of our number had an obvious coronary. There were more than a hundred physicians on the plane, all of whom felt the man should be returned to the United States. Everyone agreed—except the physician's wife, who said, "Oh, he's fine, he's just had the flu. He won't have any problems as soon as we get on our vacation. We've planned this trip for a year, and I want to go on it."

One hundred physicians responded, "You've got to go back. This plane has to return." But his wife urged him to continue, and there was little that anyone could do except feel very uncomfortable for the rest of the trip.

By the time we reached England, the patient was extremely ill and was transferred to a hospital. He managed to return to the United States, but nine months later he died.

Some families overreact to illnesses, and some under-react. We all know that people can become overwhelmed by emergency situations, but I have also found many cases where people become underwhelmed.

The medical society's memorial service was quite beautiful and was attended by a few of the physicians who were on that flight to Europe. No mention was made of the plane trip, but many of us in attendance knew the real story. I for one couldn't stop thinking about it.

Yes, a doctor is always a doctor wherever he goes—and he's always a doctor, even when he's the patient. That can be tough for both doctor and patient.

When my children were very young and I was in my thirties, we took a vacation trip to the mountains. I awoke in the motel about three o'clock in the morning with intense pain in my back. I knew immediately that I had a kidney stone. Passage of a kidney stone is such an excruciating pain that narcotic addicts have been known to mimic the condition in order to receive narcotics prescriptions from physicians. I left my family in the motel and drove to a local hospital emergency room. There was no doctor on duty, and when I described my symptoms over the phone to the doctor on call, he suspected I was just such a vacationing addict and he would not come to the hospital to see me.

Even the emergency room staff seemed to think I had a drug problem. Nothing I could do or say would convince them to get me some pain relief. They insisted that I wait until morning to be seen by a physician. Of course, I probably looked like a drug addict, with glassy, tearing eyes and a horrible grimace on my face.

Then I remembered something. I went out to my car, reached into my medical bag and found an unopened bottle of morphine sulfate. I returned to the emergency room, put the morphine bottle on the table in front of the nurse and yelled, "If I wanted narcotics, would I have this with me? Now get me a doctor!" And they did.

I do not suggest that every physician carry his own heavy narcotics when traveling, but I never knew when I might encounter someone with a coronary or injury. I kept that bottle with me, unopened, for years. It was there when I needed it in the mountains, if only for demonstration purposes. And the incident gave me more empathy for patients who sometimes justifiably feel their condition isn't being taken seriously enough.

Physicians often look out for other physicians in a very paternal and fraternal way. This sometimes makes being the patient a little easier for a doctor.

A few years after my kidney stone incident, another stone, a large one, was discovered in a distant part of my urinary tract. A condition like this required surgery and many weeks of convalescence. This would certainly have been a disaster for my medical practice. Regardless of how much rapport exists between doctor and patient, a prolonged illness in a physician frightens patients. When they hear of the doctor's illness, if they think the doctor may be unavailable to them, they will quickly ask for their records and go elsewhere.

My urologist told me about a new treatment for kidney stones called lithotripsy, which involves breaking up the stone with electronic shock waves. Although it was still in the experimental stage, this was obviously the treatment of the future for most kidney stones. No surgery was involved, and the recovery time was a few days, at most. There were only two research projects going on in the United States and the procedure was not likely to be approved by the Food and Drug Administration for quite a while. Although thousands of people all over the country were candidates for the treatment, only two people could have the procedure each day. I called some friends and was accepted as one of the test patients in Indianapolis, Indiana. I believe I learned the word for such calls in South America—it was *protección*.

At the hospital in Indianapolis, I learned that one patient would be seen at nine o'clock in the morning, with a full (and fully alert) staff, no need to fast during the day and an anticipated discharge from the hospital by afternoon. The other patient would be seen at one o'clock in the morning, with a minimal, night-shift nursing staff and would need to fast during the previous day.

It didn't take a lot of pondering to realize which was the more desirable time slot. So I was very disappointed to hear that the other patient to be seen that day, besides me, was the actor Burt Reynolds. I knew I couldn't compete.

I was in my hospital room, readying myself for a long day of reading and fasting, when I heard a knock on the door. The operating room staff came in to take me for the morning time slot.

A few days later, my hospital stay was completed and I prepared to leave. The attending physician came by on rounds, and I thanked him for giving me the morning time slot. I told him I'd expected it to be allotted to Burt Reynolds.

"I'm surprised you thought so," said the physician. "Sure, he's a movie star, but you're a doctor and we look out for our own."

Remarks like that are practically guaranteed to speed a physician-patient's recovery. I checked out of the hospital with a smile on my face. But then Burt Reynolds may have gotten a little more personal attention from the nursing staff.

While most of us are not of movie star status, we physicians do enjoy a higher-than-average rate of recognition in our communities, often in unexpected places.

Sometimes when I am writing a check at a local store, going to the barbershop for a haircut or pumping gas, people come up to me and remind me of their visits to my office. My wife and children will never admit it, but I think they are pleased to hear comments on the order of: "Your dad (or husband) got me to where I am now." My family and I appreciate this, and perhaps have become accustomed to it. To be honest, we're surprised when we're not recognized. I understand that celebrities have the same feelings. They complain that they cannot go out without people staring at them or trying to start a conversation, but they are disappointed when they are not recognized.

Sometimes a physician who has been practicing in the same community for a long time will have his dinner disturbed or have a hurried trip to the store made longer as a patient recounts his long and detailed connection. This always seems to happen to me when my car is double-parked.

There are times when being recognized can be an awkward experience. This happened to me twice recently, and in both cases I was lying prone on an operating room stretcher awaiting a surgical procedure.

On one occasion, I was going to have surgery for arthritis of the foot. Like any patient, I was anxious about the impending surgery. As I was wheeled down the hospital corridor toward the operating room, the sweet young nurse who was pushing the head of my stretcher exclaimed, "Oh, Dr. Banov, you saw my child two weeks ago with her cough, and do you know, it's still there. Do you think an antibiotic would be appropriate?"

I responded reflexively, "Well, I really don't know. It could be a lot of things. Perhaps, if I could review her records, I could give you some advice."

"Oh, you don't need the records," the nurse replied. "I can describe the cough."

The nurse talked to me about her daughter's condition all the way down the corridor. After what seemed like an hour but was probably less than a minute, we arrived in the operating room. I was relieved to see the anesthesiologist. I was sure that he would put a stop to the nurse's chatter. But he was also a patient of mine, and began to tell me about his asthma and the effects of temperature changes on his breathing. He wanted me to observe the temperature in the operating room because this was the environment that he thought was aggravating his asthma.

I'd like to think these medical professionals were trying to distract me, but they had the opposite effect. I wished with all my heart that I knew no one in the hospital or community. I simply wanted to be a patient.

On another occasion I was in my urologist's office, about to have a diagnostic cystoscopy under light general anesthesia. A cystoscopy can sometimes be uncomfortable, so an anesthesiologist came to my urologist's office. The anesthesiologist introduced herself and then put in an intravenous line. The anesthetic would drip through the line into my arm and put me to sleep. It reminded me of a television program I had seen recently, in which the condemned prisoner was about to be executed. As he was lying on the gurney, a lethal dose of medication was injected.

I roused myself from this soothing train of thought to say out loud that I appreciated the anesthesiologist making this outpatient visit. She replied, "Oh, Charles, I have waited many years to do something for you."

I thought this was a strange remark, and her explanation did not make it any less strange. She told me that I had testified some years before in a malpractice case where she was the defendant. I had been the principal expert witness.

I wondered whether my testimony had helped the defense or the plaintiff, and I was just about to ask her whose side I'd been on when I drifted off to sleep. I don't know what dark dreams I may have had, but when I woke up (and I did, fortunately, wake up), I picked up right where I'd left off. "Was my testimony helpful to you?" I asked as soon as I opened my eyes.

"It certainly was. You saved my ass."

With that reassurance, I went back to sleep.

I've noticed that I find many of my most interesting allergy cases outside of my examining room. In one dramatic instance, I was almost seventy years old and beginning to think that the practice of allergy might be getting routine.

I was having my own medical troubles—dental, this time—and was recovering in the dentist's operating room after a root canal procedure. The dentist stepped out of the room, but the dental assistant was still there.

Within a few minutes, I noticed the assistant was developing a flush and was scratching her fingernails on her arms and face. Then she broke out in hives. Her voice became raspy, and her throat tightened up in what was developing into a severe anaphylactic reaction.

The poor woman was just able to whisper that she thought it was the shrimp she had eaten at lunch when she collapsed across my lap.

There I was in the chair, with forceps and other materials hanging out of my mouth. But I jumped up and eased her into the chair, then tried with difficulty to pull the instruments out.

What I needed immediately was adrenaline, but I couldn't find any. Mouth-to-mouth resuscitation was impossible with all that equipment in my mouth. I turned the examining room upside down in my quest for adrenaline, unceremoniously dumping the contents of all of those equipment drawers. Hundreds of horrific-looking dental instruments tumbled onto the floor. I remember thinking that dentists must hide them away on purpose for fear their patients would see them and leave in a panic.

Finally I located the adrenaline bottle and administered the injection. The patient responded immediately. In fact, she was well enough to glare at me and demand to know who in hell was going to clean up this mess.

In retrospect, if there were any way that I could have transfused my own adrenaline into her, I could have avoided the search for the bottle. My pulse was racing and I was breathing like a race horse. Even though I did everything I needed to do and possibly saved this young lady's life, I was plain scared to death. The very last thing that would have crossed my mind was who would clean up the mess.

When the dentist came back into the room, he found his dental assistant in the chair. His patient, instruments falling out of his mouth, hovered over her, loading a second dose of adrenaline into a syringe. What a picture! The patient/assistant recovered completely and now avoids shrimp. The dentist seems to have recovered too.

But I'm a little more wary of dentists' offices.

Another incident that also involved anaphylaxis (a term that means a severe, potentially life-threatening allergic reaction) occurred in an even more public setting. I was asked to give a television interview on the subject of the forthcoming ragweed season. The city of Charleston is on a peninsula, and the TV studio was in Mount Pleasant, across the Cooper River. I was too busy during the day to get over to the station, so Jean Wade, the reporter who was also the show's host, arranged to tape our interview after my office hours.

Jean came by to pick me up from my office at about six o'clock one evening, and as we were getting into her car for the trip to the studio, she showed me a ragweed bush and asked if I could identify it. I confirmed that this was, indeed, ragweed. She broke off a large branch and put it in the back seat.

It was a typically warm, South Carolina fall season. The windows were up, and the air conditioning was on recirculation. We arrived at the studio within a few minutes, and the interview soon began. I described allergies in general and in particular ragweed allergy. As I talked on, I noticed that Jean's voice was getting raspy. Not only that, but her eyes were watering and she was breaking out in hives.

"For example," I said, leaning forward in my chair, "you seem to be having a classic allergic reaction right now, Jean. Are you, by any chance, allergic to ragweed?"

"No, I don't remember ever having a problem with ragweed," she said. "In fact…" Jean tried to continue, but couldn't get the words out as her throat began to close up. She'd had so much direct contact with the ragweed pollen in the car, and now on the studio set, that she was truly developing severe anaphylaxis.

I did not have my physician's bag, which held adrenaline and other resuscitative drugs that could have helped her. I whispered to Jean that we must stop the interview immediately and get to a hospital.

"Oh, no, Doctor!" she croaked. "This is exactly what I needed to show my audience!" She then turned to the camera again. "See, audience? This is what an allergic reaction is like."

As her voice got worse, so did my heart rate and anxiety level. Here we were, far from a hospital, with a life-threatening allergic emergency. This was no time for a live demonstration. It was foolhardy to continue, although I was impressed with Jean's dedication to her profession.

We continued with the interview somehow. As soon as the technician said, "That's it!" we leaped out of our seats and raced back across the river to the hospital emergency room. Jean recovered and was back on the air the next day.

Many people don't fully realize the potential of a severe allergic reaction to—well, to kill you. Medical technology has developed various tools and techniques to ward off potentially fatal reactions, but a big obstacle still exists—human error.

We can help patients become less severely allergic to such things as insect stings through desensitization. It's a process that takes time though, and before it is effective, patients are still at great risk if they are re-stung by insects to which they are extremely allergic. Many of them carry an EpiPen, an adrenaline syringe that can be self-administered, even through clothing. An EpiPen can be a life-saving device if carried at all times and, most importantly, used quickly and correctly. One of those who always carried an EpiPen was my patient, Bill.

Bill, an athletic instructor at a local college, was particularly compulsive about his adrenaline syringe. He had memorized all of the data in the information sheet, which was quite an undertaking. Perhaps it was a byproduct of his training and profession, but Bill seemed remarkably confident in his own ability to avoid an allergic disaster. I wasn't so sure.

I was seeing him in the office for a sore throat one day and decided to test him. Looking at my watch, I suddenly said, "Quick! You have been stung on the arm by a wasp and are having a life-threatening allergic reaction. What will you do?"

Bill, smirking, reached down, pulled up his trouser leg and there, neatly strapped to his leg in the most dramatic, movie-like way, was the EpiPen. He whipped off the strap, which was really a length of rubber tubing, and began to tie it around his arm, one-handed, as a tourniquet. He couldn't do it. He fumbled and struggled, and dropped the EpiPen. It was a mess. Bill was never able to get his adrenaline injected in the time window for anaphylaxis. If it had been a real allergic incident, Bill would be dead.

That's why it's not enough merely to prescribe medications for patients with severe allergies. Physicians must make sure the patient knows how to take care of himself in a crisis. And since school nurses, police officers and, of course, the parents of young patients often jump in to help without waiting for a doctor to arrive (and they're quite right to do so), they, too, need the best training and education we can provide. Fortunately, we've made great progress in that area. But there is much more to do.

In the late 1980s, I had the unique experience of being one of the first allergists to become involved in what we now call the latex allergy crisis. While I may not have seen the first few cases of this life-threatening allergy to latex, I was certainly one of the first responders to the problem and raised the alarm about the problem.

For a number of years, I had been a medical consultant for EZ-EM, a company that manufactured barium enemas for use in gastrointestinal medical diagnosis. My job was to interview by phone any physicians reporting allergic reactions of their patients to EZ-EM products. About two or three times a year, someone had a rash or other mild reaction to the materials, but other than that there were no significant problems.

All of a sudden, we began receiving many reports of patients with severe, life-threatening and, in a few documented cases, fatal reactions after certain X-ray diagnostic procedures. A few cases of possible deaths after severe reactions occurring from latex product exposures were reported to the Food and Drug Administration—but these occurred before the barium was actually administered in the procedure. As soon as a latex-tipped catheter was inserted into the patients' rectums, they would suffer a drop in blood pressure, generalized itching and laryngeal edema, or anaphylaxis. This kind of reaction often required emergency treatment, including putting a breathing tube down the throat and the administration of adrenaline.

And yet radiologists whose patients had these problems seemed not to be concerned. Whenever I called them to discuss the problem, they answered, "Oh, yes. The patient is now in the intensive care unit," not worried at all.

Then we began receiving complaints from physicians whose patients were reacting whenever latex gloves were used in a medical procedure—not just in barium enemas. Dentists reported reactions from the rubber dams used in oral surgery.

For some reason, most physicians attributed the drop in blood pressure to an idiosyncratic reaction to latex rather than an allergic one. This was a very important distinction, because the treatment was quite different. In the case of an allergic reaction, the treatment of choice is adrenaline. And without adrenaline promptly administered, the sufferer risks death.

The dimensions of this crisis seemed limitless. Physicians reported reactions to such common latex products as balloons and toys. A local surgeon developed life-threatening asthma in the middle of a procedure simply by touching the surgical rubber gloves. Another surgeon's assistant breathed in the airborne material from the gloves and had a severe reaction. Certain foods began to give similar reactions to latex intolerance. A patient might have always eaten a particular food, such as banana, without any difficulty; then, after developing a rash from latex, he would suddenly have severe reactions to bananas and other fruits.

Why would such an epidemic of allergic reaction suddenly emerge, when latex had been around for years without incident? We still don't know the answer to that question. And beyond the many physicians who reported their suspicions about the cause of the reactions, there were many more who, because latex had never posed a problem before, never made the connection. It was crucial to broadcast this information as quickly as possible. We could not afford the luxury of waiting for the usual time-consuming process of writing formal medical journal articles or developing programs of continuing medical education for physicians. It was equally important to avoid panicking people who might think they could die by handling a rubber band.

One of the fastest ways to spread new medical information is through the communication systems and public relations firms of medical supply and pharmaceutical companies.

I contacted the president of EZ-EM, locating him on a glacier in Alaska. When I described the problem, he understood immediately that this news would not be good for his company. His products relied on latex balloons to keep the barium in place during X-rays. He might also suffer from guilt-by-association—stock market investors might associate EZ-EM with negative news about latex.

He might have chosen to stall for time while he consulted with his corporate attorneys about possible liability. Instead, he advised me to contact the American College of Radiology so that they'd issue an urgent warning, and he suggested some other steps to take immediately. He understood that every minute wasted increased the possibility of lives lost.

His company did, indeed, suffer financially, but it was the right thing to do for all of us. The crisis of latex allergy is still with us. Despite all of our sophisticated medical diagnostics, we simply have not been able to isolate the antigen, or allergy-producing part of latex. For this reason, we cannot find out if a person is allergic to latex until he or she has a reaction to it. And with the widespread use of this substance in everyday life, as well as in the medical profession, the chance of reaction is huge.

For all those who are as intrigued by medical detective work as I am, I offer latex allergy at the top of the list of Unsolved Mysteries.

Chapter 9

Now It Can Be Told

I always thought I'd have made a great undercover agent—a detective, an investigator or a spy. So when it happened that I was involved in passing confidential messages via electronic eavesdropping and funding political dissidents in the Soviet Union, I wasn't entirely unhappy about it.

The year 1971 was in the middle of the cold war with the Soviet Union. Daily life was infused with political jabs and propaganda from both sides. In the midst of a national atmosphere of suspicion, I received a call from a mysterious Florida physician. I wasn't personally acquainted with him, and I had never heard of him professionally. He invited me to join a special medical mission to the Soviet Union. The stated objective of the trip was to visit and observe Soviet medical outpatient clinics. The mission was not sponsored by any organization that I was familiar with and appeared to be put together by a group of individuals about whom I knew nothing.

The Florida physician who was organizing the trip had some amazing connections in the travel industry. The cost for the trip—round-trip airfare to Moscow and then to Leningrad, all hotel and travel expenses and special travel arrangements included—would be $360 each for my wife and me. Granted, the trip would take place in the middle of the Russian winter—not exactly the height of the tourist season.

Even so, this was an unbelievable offer, and I accepted. I can't believe I was so trusting or stupid as to ask no other questions about the trip. Maybe I was afraid the bubble would burst and I would miss out on this ridiculously inexpensive opportunity. But I was so intrigued by the opportunity to visit the Soviet Union that I chose to believe it.

The arrangements grew more, not less, peculiar. There was never any written correspondence confirming plans. There were only telephone calls. The doctor was taking care of the difficult-to-obtain visas (he somehow knew that Nancy and I had active passports). Our tickets and itinerary would not be given to us until the group gathered in New York.

When we did meet in New York, I found the group even more surprising. Of the fourteen physicians in the group, I could identify only three who were true physicians. It is not always possible to tell when someone is a physician, but I can certainly tell when someone is not. One of the three true physicians was a family practitioner and part-time allergist from Wisconsin. He was as confused as I about why he was invited to join the trip. The second of the three was a surgeon from Wisconsin whom I had met briefly in my training days at Milwaukee County Hospital.

The third physician was a pathologist who was accompanied by his girlfriend. She spoke very little and seemed to disappear for hours at a time, reappearing during scheduled activities. This couple argued loudly about every possible issue, beginning with the taxicab ride to the airport. In our Moscow hotel, we could hear them scream, sometimes from passion, but more often one was beating the other. The next morning at breakfast they would have the bruises to match. Sometime after this trip, *Newsweek* would report that the pathologist had been indicted for murdering his sweetheart by giving her medication to simulate a diabetic coma.

We started off flying to Stockholm in the opulent, first-class section of Delta Airlines. We continued on to Moscow via the cold, impersonal and foul-smelling planes of Aeroflot, the Russian airline. I would have backed out any number of times each day because of concern over what we had gotten ourselves into, but I did not want to appear lacking in adventurous spirit. (Months later, in the safety of our home, Nancy confided to me that she would have backed out in a minute too, but didn't want to appear weak in my eyes.) So I proceeded along like everyone else, thinking this would be a real adventure.

As we passed a checkpoint where an armed guard in his booth raised the barrier to admit us one by one, Nancy (whose comments I often compare to Gracie Allen's), remarked, "This is just like going behind the iron curtain." I cannot imagine anything more "behind the iron curtain" than going through the last checkpoint from the west to the east in the 1970s.

Everywhere we went, the same guide, a cold and distant woman who was the epitome of Russian bureaucracy, escorted us. We were given numerous rules about what we could and could not do: remain together, sit at the same position at the table for every meal, don't talk freely with anyone on the street, strictly adhere to the Soviet government's curfews and rules. We weren't given room keys at the hotel. There was a desk and a registrar on each floor instead of just one in the lobby. After we entered our rooms, the doors were locked from the outside by the registrar.

Our schedule was rigorous. We toured a number of completely unrelated locations and activities. On one trip we might stop at a hospital clinic providing emergency service for some high-rise apartments and meet with the attending physicians there. The next visit might be to examine the structure of a bridge in which none of us non-engineers had any experience or interest. One of our "doctors," who had no more medical training than a third grader, asked the questions. His questions were invariably about highly detailed and non-medical minutiae: "How high is the second span of the bridge?" "What relationship is that to the saline content of the water?" This went on the entire time we were there. He always carried a large wall thermometer with him. Throughout the trip he would hold up the group while he went to check the outside temperature. We thought this particularly stupid. It didn't take a rocket scientist—or even a trained physician—to tell that it was cold outside during the winter in Russia. Two members of our party disappeared after the first day. Our guide didn't ask about them and no explanation was offered. One of the two showed up on the airplane at the last minute, just as we were returning to the States. We never found out what happened to the other one.

I had my own special agenda for this trip. I wanted to see for myself if the stories about the persecution of Russian Jews were true. My quest was made almost impossible by the fact that we could go nowhere without a guide, and even if we could manage to get away, none of us spoke Russian.

But the surgeon from Wisconsin also had a secret that no one, especially not the trip's organizers, knew. He could speak a little Russian. He'd picked it up during World War II and, fortunately for me, thought better of revealing this fact to our hosts.

One morning the Wisconsin surgeon and I rose very early and caught a taxi to a synagogue in a suburb of Moscow. About a dozen old men were there, making matzo for Passover. They told us in detail about the Soviet persecution of Jews. Their synagogue was allowed to remain open only as a showpiece for visitors. Had our visit been planned, they said, we would have seen quite a different picture.

We rejoined our group at breakfast. No one asked where we'd been or seemed aware at all that we had gone off by ourselves. I mentioned to our guide that I would like to see a synagogue because I had heard about a good deal of religious prejudice in the Soviet Union. She said it could be arranged for the following Saturday.

The old men were right. When we arrived at the same synagogue that Saturday, it was filled with young people. There was singing, a sermon—everyone was happy. It was the very picture of freedom of worship, but it was all a charade. I couldn't help thinking of what the Nazis had done at Theresienstadt concentration camp: a make-believe model village was constructed to convince the outside world that the poor camp inmates were happily living in a humane environment.

The synagogue visit was the highlight of my Russian adventure, but I should not have done it, as I learned a few years later while working with an organization concerned about the oppression of Soviet Jews. Those elderly gentlemen may have put themselves at great risk by telling us what they did. They took that risk hoping that we would do something with the information, but I was not an official representative of any government and I had no role in any group that could help them. I did nothing but recount this story to friends and family over the years. I only hope that my later efforts on their behalf made up for any negative consequences of my visit.

Even in medical situations, I saw tyranny and oppression at work in the Soviet Union. We were taken to a premier hospital for children. In a group of apparently healthy children who were there for evaluation of heart murmurs, I saw a child with obvious Down's syndrome. I asked if the retarded children were mainstreamed. The head physician said, "We do not have retardation in the Soviet Union. Down's syndrome? It is very rare, and I didn't see the child you mentioned." I asked if we could see those children again so that I could point out the child. When we went back to the ward less than an hour later, the same children were there, except for the one with Down's syndrome. It was very important at that time for the Soviets to present the perfect society, without any visible flaws. It was a chilling echo of Adolph Hitler.

Soviet medical care, it turned out, was an inexplicable blend of up-to-date research and equipment and out-of-date systems and protocols. For example, after childbirth they kept the mothers on bed rest for seven to ten days. There were marvelous, sophisticated, tertiary-care hospitals with the latest equipment, but the vast majority of medical care was given by poorly trained, inexperienced nurse practitioners. Although the Soviets kept careful accounting of medical expenditures (which they showed us), the allocation of those resources was purely political.

Of course, if I had wanted to let them know my opinion of their medical system, all I had to do was whisper it to Nancy in our hotel room. Our rooms were thoroughly bugged, as I found out one morning. I looked in the mirror to shave and saw a small electronic device looking back at me. If one of us asked a question in the seclusion of our room, the guide would answer it the next morning at breakfast. We got into the habit of writing notes to each other. I came to cherish the assumption of privacy in America that, before this trip, I'd taken for granted.

In spite of the clear message from the Soviet government and our tour leaders to obey the rules and accept on its face the picture of Soviet society as presented to us, I couldn't stop thinking and wondering about the Soviet dissidents we Westerners had heard about. For a variety of reasons, including religious persecution, they tried to leave the country and were denied the opportunity. The very act of applying for an exit visa had, essentially, ruined their lives. These professionals from all occupations were relegated to menial jobs.

On our third night in Moscow, I contracted food poisoning. Unfortunately, it was the night our group was going to attend a performance of the Bolshoi Ballet. Nancy decided to go with the group, and I stayed behind in our hotel room. A few hours later, when I was feeling better, I decided to join the group at the ballet. That's how I found out that our hotel room doors were locked from the outside. With enough banging on the door and shouted threats, I was released and found a driver to take me to the theater. My official guide was nowhere about. Thinking I was safely locked in, he'd probably taken an unauthorized coffee break.

By then, everyone had left the theater. Nancy and another couple from the group had gone on to a restaurant for an evening snack. When I finally caught up with her at the restaurant, she told me she had met a group of "dissidents" at a bookstore. She introduced me to Sergei, a biochemical engineer who had been relegated to a job tending a boiler in a large apartment house. Sergei was meeting some of his colleagues later that night and asked us if we would like to join them. I do not know what possessed me to go with this stranger, but the desire to meet Russian dissidents was overwhelming.

We met in the basement boiler room of a large apartment building. In very broken English, Sergei told us about how they could not speak in public to Americans or to any strangers. They got their news from the BBC. They survived the austerity of the Soviet economy through the black market, a necessary, albeit dangerous, fact of life for those emotionally imprisoned people.

I foolishly gave this group a contribution of one hundred American dollars.

The Soviets exerted fanatical control over foreign currency. When one entered the Soviet Union, the amount of money brought in was counted to the penny, and upon leaving, every penny spent had to be accounted for with receipts. Just before we were to leave the country, I realized I'd have to explain why I could not produce this money and did not have a receipt for purchases to account for the missing money. A wise foreigner in Moscow gave me some advice that ultimately kept me out of trouble: I went to a bar near the hotel where American dollars could be spent, and pretended that I was drinking quite a bit. When my bar tab reached $100, I asked for a receipt and pretended to stagger out. The Soviets accepted my explanation that I truly loved their vodka.

To this day, we do not know what actually took place on that trip. But some things we do know. There were at least one or two people in our group whom our American intelligence agencies were using for information gathering. Perhaps it was that annoying man who kept asking the ridiculously minute questions: if he became known for asking unrelated and foolish questions, perhaps he could slip in a few important questions without arousing suspicion and actually receive answers. Maybe it was the leader, who left the group for a few days. Or maybe it was the couple who disappeared the first day, with only one of them reappearing just before departure time. Maybe it was all of them! The only thing we are certain of is that it wasn't us (although when you are in that environment for a while, you begin to wonder about yourself). The entire trip was set up so that these agents could be allowed to observe what was going on in the Soviet Union. We were fillers, extras in this real-life spy movie. Well, I'd always loved the movies.

In October 1962, the United States of America became involved in one of the most serious political and military confrontations in its history—the Cuban missile crisis. For me, this was not simply a paragraph in a history book or a news article clipped from the daily paper. I was there. (And I was also a little bleary-eyed, as Nancy and I then had three children under the age of five.)

President John F. Kennedy had announced the existence of missiles in Cuba provided by the Soviet Union and capable of striking the continental United States. Two days later, three B-52 bombers landed at Charleston's civilian airport next to the air force base. These were Strategic Air Command (SAC) planes, which, as everyone knew, carried our major nuclear retaliatory weapons. We wanted to avoid the errors of Pearl Harbor, where our aircraft had been packed neatly together on military bases. The deployment of these planes, either in the air or at small, non-SAC bases such as Charleston, was the last stage before all-out thermonuclear war. By all indications we were truly "eyeball to eyeball" with the Soviets and their surrogates, the Cubans. We were on the brink of war.

The next morning I received a telephone call at five o'clock from the Charleston Naval Hospital, urgently requesting that I assemble a group of internal medicine specialists or general practitioners with some experience with cardiology who could take over the care of a group of very ill patients at the hospital.

In the preparations for war and the expectation of unprecedented numbers of casualties, and in the massive deployment of forces to Florida in anticipation of a Cuban invasion, no one had made plans for the disposition of the many critically ill patients already at the naval hospital. The hospital's doctors were being sent to marine combat units, and no replacements had been identified. There were simply no medical professionals left at the hospital to care for the patients.

I was a civilian consultant to the naval hospital, a position that, most days, demanded little of me. Through my contact with Dr. William Lukash, chief of gastroenterology at the hospital and with whom I studied for my specialty board exams (and who became the personal physician to two U.S. presidents), I was called that morning to help with a desperate situation. The hospital's beds were filled with elderly retired veterans who had chosen to live in Charleston to be close to the naval hospital. That meant that there were more truly ill patients than most hospitals of that size might handle.

I called a number of my colleagues in the community and explained the situation. They, like me, had full patient schedules, concern about malpractice potential and some had been trying to retire. Even so, not one refused to help. They all came in, and they all were desperately needed. Years later, in the aftermath of the decimation caused by Hurricane Katrina, I called upon my colleagues in Charleston to help obtain much-needed drugs from the pharmaceutical representatives when the national relief organizations fell short. In both of these situations, governmental agencies failed to provide appropriate distribution of physicians. Even after the secrets of the Cuban mis sile crisis were all told, I have not seen any revelations about the sudden withdrawal of physicians from their critically ill patients during a national emergency.

Some secrets of the cold war remain.

Sometimes the stress of those cold war years came out in other ways. Once I found myself in the middle of a bizarre incident so improbable that I never would have believed the tale if it hadn't happened to me.

I had only been in practice about a month. I was locking up the office after seeing patients on a Saturday morning when a very distraught, well-dressed patient banged on my door yelling, "Is the doctor in? Is the doctor in?"

"I'm the doctor," I replied. "How can I help you? Did another doctor refer you to me?"

"I don't know what kind of doctor you are. I came into Charleston from the naval base, and I need to see a doctor— any doctor—right away."

I asked him what his problem was, and he insisted that I must first lock the door. He asked if I was sure that no one else could hear us. Obviously I had a paranoid, mentally ill man on my hands. I tried to figure out how I could get free to call for help. Who knew what this person might do in his condition?

When the doors were locked and the window shades drawn, he told me his story.

"I'm a civilian," he said, "a chief engineer with the navy. I help design nuclear submarines and missile carriers. I've just come back from a test cruise in the most advanced nuclear sub ever developed." His position required psychiatric evaluations and follow-up, not to mention security clearances. He showed me his identification and papers. The more I talked to this man, the more I realized that every word he said was true. He was not at all mentally ill, but under a tremendous strain.

"I feel like I'm on the edge of a crackup. I need a rest, Doc, but I know too much. After what happened with the recent spy trials and exposés, if I admit how I'm feeling, my career will be over. Not only that, if the navy doesn't lock me up, the government will be watching every move I make for the rest of my life, believe me."

I believed him, but I doubted that anyone else would. I realized that this man, with the information he carried, would be of invaluable help to our enemies, and therefore an ideal kidnap candidate. I was very concerned. If I called the local police or the FBI, they probably would just send him right back to the navy, where he was sure he should not go. And I wasn't sure what this might do to the navy's—or any security agency's—opinion of me, no matter how accidental I knew my involvement to be. I'd probably end up sharing a mental ward with my new patient.

My thinking was getting a bit paranoid, in tandem with that of my patient. But the atmosphere of the times fostered suspicion, even of our own government, regardless of our constitutional rights.

Things got worse: the man began to suffer a severe anxiety attack, with a true psychotic panic. I had no nursing staff with me and I was alone in the office, but I gave him an intravenous sedative, and he promptly went to sleep on my sofa. I locked the doors every way I could and tried to keep pinching myself to make sure that this wasn't some dream after a Saturday afternoon B-movie.

Then I had an idea that proved to be my salvation. I called one of my patients, a boyhood friend who was now a local FBI agent. Because he knew me to be a reasonable person, he believed my story. Within an hour, three agents came to the office, and I turned my patient over to them. Officially, I never learned what happened. Unofficially, the man wrote me a note with two words on it: Thank you. He delivered this letter in person. Shortly after his visit I received a beautiful photograph, which had been security cleared, of one of the newest submarines in our fleet, as a gift for my son. I could not tell that story until after the fall of the Soviet Union in 1991.

There were other times when the cold war, or its side effects, invaded the homefront. In the 1980s, we still were very concerned about the power and instability of the Soviet Union, and Charleston, with its naval base and shipyard, was the homeport for much of our submarine nuclear force.

I was still a consultant to the navy, and so received another urgent call from the naval hospital. One of our most advanced nuclear submarines had recently embarked on a two-month deployment to an undisclosed part of the world. The wife of a crewmember had become ill; she might have been coming down with chicken pox. This would not seem on the surface to be a major crisis for the navy. But her husband, apparently, had never been exposed, and surprisingly, a number of the male crew, according to their naval health records, had never had chicken pox. The navy was looking at the very real possibility of an epidemic of chicken pox on a nuclear submarine in the middle of the cold war.

There was at least one clear solution to the problem—bring the sub back to port. But things are never that simple in the navy. In those days, communication with these vessels was one way. When on a mission, the sub could receive messages but could not break radio silence by responding. Chicken pox in adults is far more severe than in children, and if there were an outbreak onboard, naval command would not be able to help. Even more critical, recalling the sub would create a hole in the country's nuclear defense network. Every resource, from the Strategic Air Command on down, would have to be redirected at huge expense, not to mention difficulty and confusion.

The naval command needed to know if the crewman's wife was in the early stages of chicken pox. Not only had I never seen an adult case of chicken pox, but I was not trained to diagnose its early stages in an adult. This was one hell of a responsibility to thrust upon a non-active-duty navy physician.

I called my infectious disease consultant at the Medical University of South Carolina, as well as two pediatricians with whom I had professional relationships, but none of them could help me. When chicken pox is fully developed, there's no question about what it is, but an early diagnosis is difficult to make. The poor woman was shuttled by ambulance from one physician to another, while I updated the Bureau of Medicine and Surgery every thirty minutes.

The experts were evenly divided: half thought they were seeing early-stage chicken pox, and the other half thought not. The final decision rested with me. I recalled the submarine.

The next morning, the crewman's wife was covered with the unmistakable blisters of chicken pox, and when the submarine arrived back in port, there were, indeed, several cases onboard. I don't know how much it cost the navy to recall that ship, either in dollars or defense, and I don't care. I'm just glad I made the right decision.

The intersection with the Soviet Union happened in many areas of my life in those days. I was president of the Charleston Jewish Welfare Committee and very involved in helping Jews leave Russia, where they were persecuted because of their religion. Soviet Jews came to many communities in America and we adopted some of them into our community in Charleston. They were hard workers, and did any job offered them. I was very interested in their conditions in the Soviet Union. Had they really been mistreated, or was their coming to our country more a matter of economics than of religion? Why did they all not go to Israel? Many would simply go to Israel to get out of Russia and then would come to the United States. Were they honest about their reasons for leaving Russia?

Through my involvement with the Jewish community of Charleston, I was invited to a briefing from Thomas G., then a senior representative of the American Bar Association, who had been chosen as an independent observer to evaluate the treatment of religious groups in the Soviet Union. He was not Jewish and presumably would be completely impartial. He told his listeners the following story, which was validated by his co-presenter, an ex-CIA agent.

On the airplane leaving the United States, Thomas and his two staff members met a very delightful, newly married couple on their way to Moscow as tourists. The couple chose this honeymoon trip because the husband was newly employed by the State Department and thought this would be good experience. Significantly, his wife spoke Russian. Thomas thought her skill would be of great help to him in finding out what was really going on within the tightly controlled Soviet Union.

On the other hand, Thomas knew that if this couple were to travel with him, they would quickly be identified by Soviet intelligence, which could be disastrous for the young husband's career. He might be blacklisted from returning to work in the Soviet Union. A moral dilemma ensued: should they befriend this young couple and use them to get information or, recognizing that this would be dangerous for them, simply drop the acquaintance? After careful consideration, Thomas G. decided to befriend this young couple while in Russia.

Together, Thomas, his staff and the young couple visited private homes where tourists could not normally go. They saw (and heard, with the newlywed translators) how oppressive the old Soviet Union was and how persecuted religion was in Russia at that time. The frightening stories were all true.

The observation team used the couple, indeed: they paid for dinners, provided transportation and hotels. They spent the entire two-week trip in one another's company.

Back in the United States, Thomas was called to Washington for a formal debriefing. He asked the couple to attend. In addition, the CIA and other governmental agencies were there, as well as an Israeli Mossad officer. As he came into the room, the Israeli introduced himself and exclaimed, "Oh, I see you've met our two Mossad agents."

That chance meeting between the young couple and the representative of the American Bar Association had been well orchestrated in advance. The Israelis as well as the Jewish religious leadership in America wanted to be certain that this independent observer was given an opportunity to meet people who could show him the reality of the situation in the Soviet Union at that time. The observer, as he told us the story, added that in his opinion, all parties to the trip had been "well used."

And it answered my question: apparently the refuseniks were sincere in their desire to leave Russia for reasons other than economic. As I drove home that night, I reflected on the interesting way each of the parties in this tale had used each other. I appreciate a good O. Henry story, and this tale seemed like a good one. But the story wasn't finished.

A few years later—this time during my presidency of the American College of Allergy—I was invited by Pfizer Pharmaceutical Company to the President's Forum, which is a meeting for the exchange of ideas between the various presidents of all of the national medical societies. The forum always invited interesting speakers. This time it was an ex-KGB agent who had defected to the West.

After the lecture, I told him gleefully how we ordinary people had outfoxed the KGB and how the fact-finding committee of the American Bar Association had used the Israelis who, in turn, used them. I explained to the Russian ex-spook and KGB graduate that were he an American, he would have agreed that this was a good O. Henry story.

The man smiled. He remarked that a good KGB agent would naturally know the enemy's literature: he agreed that this was, indeed, a good O. Henry story. Then he proceeded to tell me his version of the story. This man claimed that he not only remembered hearing about the visitors I mentioned; he said that he was assigned to make sure that both groups saw exactly what the Soviets wanted them to see. Furthermore, he claimed that the KGB knew in advance that Mossad had arranged for the young travelers to meet. According to his version, while the observer and Mossad both thought they had outfoxed the Soviets, the Soviets were outfoxing them. Who knows the real version?

This I do know: O. Henry was probably enjoying the whole show from his front-row seat in heaven.

In the late 1990s, after the collapse of the Soviet Union, I made another trip to Russia, this time as an invited speaker. By then, the country was in financial decline and organized crime was flourishing. It happened that the Russian mafia often sponsored scientific meetings in Russia. These gangsters managed to have legitimate professional and social functions, such as conventions, brought to large Russian cities, and they provided the honoraria for international speakers. The hotel business, transportation and all the other profits from conventions slipped back into the hands of these thugs. One always knew when the invitation came indirectly from the Russian mafia: the honoraria were always paid in crisp $100 bills left in an envelope on the bed.

On one of these speaking trips, in 1998, I was asked to lecture on cat allergy. I don't know if there are any scientific studies to back me up, but I've observed that those who love cats the most are the most allergic to them. I have had the unpleasant duty of advising patients to give away their cats; it's like asking a parent to put up a child for adoption. In the 1980s, researchers proved that cat allergy is caused by the dander of the cat. Allergy sufferers are more allergic to male cats than to female cats because the allergic material in the dander and saliva of the cat is hormone-related. In many cases, castration of the cat helps to decrease the cat's allergic effect, and many cat lovers have been able to tolerate their cats despite their allergy to them. This was a major breakthrough in environmental control for asthmatic patients.

The meeting was held in the Kremlin. More than a thousand Russian physicians were invited by sponsoring pharmaceutical companies. The audience was given a dinner and unlimited vodka. When it came time for me to give my lecture, I found myself facing an unruly, anti-American audience more interested in commenting on the recent Monica Lewinsky affair than on my scientific presentation. Many ribald remarks were made about President Bill Clinton and his indiscretions. Regardless of my political feelings, it was very uncomfortable to have these Russians insult America this way, and after almost an hour of watching my audience bang on the tables with their shoes, a la Khrushchev, and hearing rude jokes about the United States, I'm afraid I got angry.

I asked the projectionist to put the first slide up to begin the lecture. Unfortunately, the first slide's headline read: "If the cat becomes intolerable, CASTRATE him." The audience screamed with laughter, assuming I was joining in the Lewinsky joke. I could only stand there with a Jack Benny expression on my face and think to myself that we were foolish to worry about these people acting so stupidly for almost fifty years. In fact, when I received my post-lecture assessment, I had the highest grade for my "humorous" presentation.

If those Russian physicians never figured out how to help their allergic patients it was their own damn fault.

Cat allergy, though, is serious business. Often we simply are unable to separate the beloved cat and allergic owner. We then have no alternative but to give the patient allergy shots to build up her immunity to the cat. Recently, after explaining the process in great detail to a patient, she came back the following week for her first allergy shot carrying her cat in her arms. My entire office—crowded waiting room, receptionists and assistants—erupted. The patient was rushed back to my office for a stern lecture on the inappropriateness of taking a cat into an allergist's office.

"But, Doctor," said the patient, "if I don't bring Ginger in with me, how will she receive her allergy shot?" Perhaps she should be forgiven her ignorance. Her PhD was only in nuclear physics.

Chapter 10

Hurricanes and Bioterrorism
Doctor First, Old Man Last

I've been in emergency medical situations many times during my career. Almost always, these emergencies involve only one patient at a time. On a few occasions, I was that patient.

But in 1989 I found myself in the middle of a mass emergency by the name of Hurricane Hugo. We had plenty of warning about Hugo—the storm had been coming toward us for a few days and had already caused massive damage to parts of Puerto Rico and some Caribbean islands. Savannah was evacuated, but then the storm changed course and headed north. It was due to hit Charleston about twenty-four hours after the government began to evacuate the Lowcountry. I felt guilty evacuating with the rest of my family and decided to see if I could be of some help in the coming storm.

Our daughter Pamela had been living at the Coastal Residential Center since age thirteen (she was then twenty-three), so I understood that the staff and their residents would need extra help. I offered to come over and pitch in—change diapers, do cleanup or whatever job needed doing. This way I could also keep an eye on my daughter should storm conditions get really bad.

There was a full-time pediatrician at the center, and although I worried that an allergist would just be in the way during a real medical emergency—how often does

MEDEVAC or the highway patrol need to be concerned about a wheeze, sneeze or itch when people's roofs are being blown off?—I hoped I could be at least another pair of reliable hands in any medical situation.

Earlier in the day, Nancy left for Columbia with my octogenarian parents. Columbia was well inland and, we thought, would be spared the power of the storm. I put on my jeans and work shirt, drove to the Coastal Center and promptly got caught in a traffic jam of unbelievable proportions.

By the time I arrived at the center, the first civilians had arrived. (We referred to anyone who was neither a client nor a staff member at the center—an area resident, for example— as a civilian.) I was assigned to a building adjacent to the center that was normally used for recreational purposes. There, huddling together, even though the temperature was mild, were about seventy-five refugees from the surrounding community. The wind was howling, rain falling and lashing the buildings horizontally. We tried to relax everyone, particularly the children, with songs and stories. If nothing else, it helped pass the time.

Before long, a young woman arrived, helped in by her husband, in real distress. She was twenty-six years old, with one small child, and in her first trimester of pregnancy. Within the past few hours, since the storm began, she'd developed increasing abdominal pain. By the time she arrived at the Coastal Center, she was screaming in agony. Her belly was rigid and tight. It was clear to me that she was either miscarrying or suffering from a tubal pregnancy that was about ready to rupture or had already ruptured. Her blood pressure began dropping precipitously. This was a real medical emergency if there ever was one.

Meanwhile, the storm was making so much noise that even in a closed building we could not hear each other and resorted to using crude sign language. We had not even reached the midpoint of the eye. Our phones were still working, and I called every medical facility I could reach, including the naval hospital. But the highway patrol, when I finally got through, told me it might be as long as eighteen hours before anyone could get through all of the fallen trees. Massive old oaks had been knocked over like toothpicks, making the highways impassable.

Of the medical professionals who had volunteered to remain at the center, the pediatrician and the senior nurse, neither had had much surgical experience. None of the three of us knew if the woman's rigid belly signified a tubal pregnancy. All of us knew that a tubal pregnancy, if left to rupture without emergency surgery, could be fatal. Were we morally obligated to attempt surgery? I thought back to World War II movies, where appendectomies were performed in submarines under enemy waters. Conditions here were just about as bad. We could give spinal anesthesia, but not blood transfusion. I had Demerol in my bag that could relieve her pain, but it might aggravate the shock. Certainly it would mask further examination should we be able to locate a gynecologist. It looked like it would be up to me to make the decision.

As we were trying to decide what to do, and the woman continued to scream in pain, the roof fell in—literally. I followed the sounds of yells and more screams to discover four people holding up the metal roof with broomsticks.

Then the infirmary called. Another civilian had been brought in from town with severe shortness of breath. I ran to the infirmary to examine my new patient, who was obviously in pulmonary edema caused by heart failure. Fortunately, I did have some diuretics and cardiovascular drugs in my black bag, past their expiration date but still able to give rather dramatic relief to the poor fellow. I spent the night running back and forth between my patients.

It seemed to take forever, but finally the highway patrol broke through. The wind was still raging, but most of the roofs held. Both of my patients held on, too. The young woman was taken to the naval hospital, where immediate surgery was performed for a tubal pregnancy rupture. The heart patient survived as well. I spent the rest of the day praying and, after it was over, before dawn, slept deeply.

I realized that I was wrong about an allergist's potential for helping in a natural disaster. An allergist has many things to offer that are rather unique to his specialty: formal training in both pediatrics and internal medicine; experience with pulmonary complications of exposure to noxious materials; extensive training and experience in immunological aspects of major environmental holocausts; the ability to see large numbers of new patients rapidly and efficiently; and familiarity with current antibiotics, bacterial resistance in epidemics and current immunization procedures.

Hugo was the worst natural disaster to hit South Carolina in a hundred years. The aftermath was expensive and lengthy. Our senator, my onetime patient Fritz Hollings, called the Federal Emergency Management Administration "a bunch of bureaucratic jackasses."

Some things don't change.

Sixteen years later, I had another opportunity to demonstrate what an allergist can do.

While Hugo was formidable and turned out to be the second-most-costly hurricane then to have hit the United States, Katrina and her sister, Rita, far surpassed it in financial loss and cost of lives. Katrina, the hurricane, devastated New Orleans and Gulf Coast cities on August 29, 2005. Katrina, the aftermath, continued to generate chaos and illness for many more months.

Like most Americans, my immediate reaction to the news of Katrina was disbelief that this devastation could occur here at home, instead of some third-world location. So many people, displaced persons in our own country, needed help. And I realized they'd need more than my sympathy and checkbook.

I called everywhere to volunteer my services, from New Orleans to our local shelters to my colleagues in neighboring states. I spent a day at Red Cross headquarters learning the "rules of volunteerism," which, if followed, would only have added to the growing bureaucratic nightmare that plagued the recovery efforts. Nevertheless, there appeared to be enough initial physician support in the first few days, and I was not called upon. All I could do was sit and listen to the news reports.

On the sixth day after the hurricane, I received a desperate call from the Texas Medical Association: "We need help now!"

Among all the physicians between Charleston and the Texas/Louisiana border, none was available to come immediately—within hours—to a remote area that had been overlooked by all the computers and all the relief organizations: San Augustine, Texas.

After the disaster in New Orleans, the governor of Texas had arranged with his counterpart in Louisiana to send a few busloads of the neediest evacuees to a well-supplied facility that was far away from the storm damage. On these buses were children with retardation from group homes and a residential center, patients with terminal disease from a hospice facility and some elderly people rescued without their usual caretakers. Included in this group, somehow, were recovering addicts and a few prisoners from flooded-out prisons.

The slow, bumper-to-bumper caravan had just reached San Augustine when the buses ran out of gas. The passengers had little water and no food, except what they had carried from the shelters in Louisiana. Then, shortly after they arrived in this little town, Hurricane Rita hit.

In the middle of the storm, the evacuees left the buses and took refuge in local churches. Most had fled New Orleans without their medications. Several diabetics had no insulin. Many of them had been exposed to foul water from the fractured levees. An epidemic of gastrointestinal infection was beginning.

Before I could help, I had to get to San Augustine. That turned out to be a major maneuver in itself. The town was sixty miles away from the nearest airport. It was quite an isolated community, smaller than Beeville and bigger (but not much bigger) than Pettus. At first, I was told that an air force plane would fly me to the nearest landing field available. I was to wait at my home for a pickup. Later, I was told that the navy was assigned the task of getting essential emergency workers to key flight destinations. Unfortunately, apparently no one told the navy.

A few days earlier, the Red Cross in Charleston had opened some well-stocked shelters to receive some survivors from New Orleans. As providers waited at the local airport for hurricane victims to arrive, we learned that the air force had inadvertently taken them to Charleston, West Virginia—there being no reason, in the midst of disaster, why the usual military snafu should not occur. I finally took a commercial flight to Shreveport, Louisiana, using that time to brush up on my obstetrics. The flight attendant was a little concerned when she saw me balancing a textbook on one knee and practicing suture knots on the seat in front of me.

At Shreveport, the sheriff's deputy picked me up and drove me to San Augustine. The gasoline shortage almost caught up with the deputy's car, but we eventually coasted into San Augustine on fumes.

Eight people had already died from the unknown gastrointestinal infection. The Centers for Disease Control tried to identify the offending organisms, but there was so much contamination in the food, water and air it was only surprising that more had not died. A lone emergency room physician had been with the group. He had found the caravan and stuck by them for three days, but then, utterly exhausted, left the area just as I arrived.

I tried to assess the resources. There was an eighteen-bed hospital in the area, already packed to capacity—patients needing admission for some type of emergency were advised to bring their own mattresses. Meals and drinking water were brought in by the National Guard. A few generators were available for people dependent upon mechanical or electrical health devices.

What we didn't have, and needed desperately, was medication, including intravenous fluid replacements. Many of the evacuees developed asthma from the contaminated water; some of the asthma medications were quite expensive and hard to come by. I called my office and explained the situation to my staff. They immediately went to work contacting local pharmaceutical representatives and my colleagues in the state. We emptied their sample closets.

The local leaders warned me that there were no sleeping facilities for any of the volunteers, but that we were welcome to use the floor of the local jail, which we did for the first night. After that, we were more comfortable using the hospital kitchen floor, if only psychologically; it was just as hard as the jail floor.

I had failed to tell our host that I was in my mid-seventies. (I contend that no one ever asked.) So when the sheriff took a look at me, he immediately offered to put me up in his home. He failed to tell me, however, that he already had each room in his home occupied by various relief workers from the town, as well as a few nurses volunteering from other communities. This was indeed a unisex experience: bathrooms and the occasional shower were in such demand that modesty was the last thing that occurred to anyone at that time.

We struggled through mistakes and lack of foresight. Although the major pharmaceutical companies had donated millions of dollars' worth of medications for the relief of hurricane victims, they were all delivered to major cities, such as New Orleans and Houston. On the second day I was there, when things were really desperate, the Red Cross called to say that they had a major delivery for us: twenty-five thousand sandwiches. What I really needed was insulin and antibiotics. I could have done without the sandwiches.

But my phone call to my office produced something of a miracle: our nursing staff was able to commandeer the necessary transportation to bring us lifesaving drugs within twenty-four hours.

Finally, five days after my arrival, when things were getting under control, we heard that the Mayo Clinic would send in physicians and support staff. Unfortunately, they, like other sources of medical supply, needed preparation time, but the situation could not wait. I'm grateful that I was able to drop everything and rush to meet the immediate need. By the time the Mayo group arrived, I was able to close all the shelters. We had made arrangements for evacuees to be housed in other, more suitable facilities.

These people had suffered. A number of them did not know where their families were. Three couples had no idea about the fate of their young children. A few young women had been raped in shelters in New Orleans. They would bear physical and emotional scars for the rest of their lives. For me, the experience brought back memories of Hugo, and also of Pettus at the beginning of my medical career. I do not know how many lives I may actually have saved in 1957, but I do know many were saved this time.

Hugo and Katrina taught me many things about myself. For example, I found it very difficult to triage, or decide which patients should receive immediate attention and which were in such bad shape that we shouldn't expend efforts to save them. I did not like the feeling of playing God in that way. I know that there are situations when triage is utterly necessary, and it is probably always a painful task for whoever must do it. In some cases, it is the only way to quickly manage hospital beds and medical facilities with great elasticity and without compromising quality of care. But as I discovered, it's hard to make the decisions.

Several months later, in May 2006, with the experience of Katrina fresh in my memory, I took up an offer to attend a training program in Israel on just how to organize help and effectively muster available medical care under extreme natural disaster or bioterrorism conditions. Regrettably, Israel has had, and continues to find, vast opportunity to improve their methods of care.

We were a group of nine surgeons, pathologists, internists and allergists/immunologists. We worked diligently all week on mannequins, well-trained actors who could simulate injuries and sophisticated equipment for detection and elimination of poisonous gas, and applying triage. At the end of the week, we participated in a graduation ceremony and were inducted into the Israel Defense Forces as reserve physicians who could come to Israel in time of need to assist in the medical community. Usually, when people work together under such stressful conditions, they form a bond. When they separate, they all hope to see one another again. After this course, as our group departed, each of us looked at the other with the same thought: may we never have to meet again as a group.

Anyone with a career in medicine is forever riding what seems like an emotional seesaw regarding the state of the profession. One day a miraculous breakthrough in research is announced. Soon after, some new therapy proves useless—or worse, dangerous. Managed care and Byzantine health insurance regulations make medical practices more complex than a rocket launch. Yet modern clinical care can improve the quality of life for thousands of very sick patients.

But every time I get discouraged, I like to think about the real triumphs—for example, the eradication of poliomyelitis. As a child, I can remember fellow grammar school students being paralyzed from the neck down with this horrible disease; others couldn't participate in sports because they were dependent on leg braces and crutches.

A patient who was paralyzed and unable to breathe spontaneously was placed in a machine called an iron lung, which created a vacuum that pumped air in and out of the lungs, and essentially breathed for him. A polio victim might spend the rest of his life in this tank, which was a depressing thought. Every child who grew up in the 1930s and '40s knew about polio and had some contact with a paralyzed person. Everyone knew about iron lungs. I remember photographs of large rooms with dozens of iron lungs, each one looking like a small submarine, in which the patient had to lie on his back twenty-four hours a day.

As a resident physician at Charity Hospital in the 1950s, there was still a ward of more than one hundred polio patients in iron lungs. I tried to develop a slide projector for one patient who was paralyzed from the neck down and could only look at the ceiling and blink his eyes. I worked out a machine with the Louisiana State University engineers' office that projected an image of the page of a book onto the ceiling. The patient turned the book's pages using his eyelids. I don't remember the details of the mechanism but we had some type of an on-off switch that required three or four squeezes of the eye to operate it. We had to make it work with more than one blink or it would go on and off constantly and defeat its purpose. It didn't do everything, but it helped a lot of people pass the time. This was an amazing breakthrough, and everyone in the ward was able to benefit from this one device.

Years later, one cold, rainy day, I had a light afternoon in the office and wanted to work in the Medical University Library across the street. In the hall of the library an iron lung was on display. I went back across the street to my office and called to my well-trained, up-to-date nursing staff. I thought it would be a good opportunity for them to see an iron lung, since most of them were too young to have seen one in use.

I asked the group, "Wouldn't you like to see an iron lung? You rarely ever see these anymore, and there is a museum piece across the way." Every one of the nurses and technicians looked at me in amazement and said, "An iron lung? What's that?"

It almost brought tears to my eyes. To this generation of medical professionals, polio was ancient history. The disease had been essentially eradicated, and fifty years later, no one—not even a nurse or technician—knew what an iron lung was; they had not even heard the term. I like to imagine that not too many years hence, I will see a patient with cancer and say to my staff, "By the way, I saw a lymphoma patient," and a well-trained person will look at me quizzically and say, "You saw a what?"

One of the horrors that medical students of my generation remember is the final moments of patients with advanced syphilis. Syphilis was very prominent in the pre-antibiotic era and is still present with us today. It was said that syphilis had so many victims that, as stated in most textbooks, "To know syphilis is to know diseases." In other words, syphilis presented signs and symptoms of just about any disease.

Often, years after an active infection with syphilis, a patient suffered either severe brain damage or damage to the blood vessels. This insidious damage could take twenty to thirty years to form. It was common to have on the wards a number of patients with syphilis of the aortic valve. Today, some things can be done for patients with this disease, so expectation of rupture is not the norm. But at that time nothing could be done. The aortic vessel was certain to rupture, spurting up blood from the patient almost to the ceiling. It was dramatic and horrible. No one who witnessed such an end could eradicate it from his dreams. Rather than upset the rest of the ward (many of whom had the same condition), the patient was given what was called an aneurysm jacket: a canvas, constrictive jacket to hold the blood in when the aorta eventually ruptured.

Almost as traumatic as seeing an aortic rupture was witnessing the moment when the nurses gave the aneurysm jacket to an advanced-stage patient. It was like pronouncing a death sentence or leading someone to a firing squad. The nurses tried to disguise what was going on, but the patients knew. Everyone on the ward knew, and certainly the patient receiving the jacket knew.

It is another one of those things that has passed with the years, and good riddance.

The last time I sat down to philosophize and evaluate the career of medicine was when I wrote a letter to my sons, Mark and Michael, when they each graduated from medical school. The words came easily because they came from my heart. Their graduations were only a few years apart, and the letters to each of them were almost identical.

> *Dear Son:*
>
> *It seems like only yesterday that I wrote you a note just before you started medical school. Actually, it seems also like yesterday when I wrote you a good luck note before you started the first grade and again when you began college. I also remember wishing you good luck when you first went to camp, when you went on your first date and when you played in your first basketball game. It seems that Mom and I always had the pleasure of wishing you good luck on some project or on some accomplishment. Your graduation from medical school beats them all.*
>
> *A physician father has no greater compliment than that of seeing his child follow along in medicine. I imagine that some of the pride comes from the pleasure of knowing that perhaps I set a good example and gave medicine a shiny face. Still, I think it is much more than that. I think that physician parents, despite their complaints, feel that there is no better career than medicine, so I think we are simply happy that you will be happy. I feel that with only one life to spend there is nothing finer than the career of medicine. I know this sounds corny, and typical parental lecturing, but, honestly, I believe it sincerely.*
>
> *Despite the complaints that we all have about the frustrations of medicine, the many changes that the field is undergoing and the legitimate criticism of some of our fellow physicians, this is*

undoubtedly the most honorable profession that has ever existed. You have always been concerned about morality and ethics, and your interest in religion and even the choice of your college major has indicated that you will only be happy in the field where you are performing good works. In my judgment, medicine is the quintessence of religiosity. Whereas religious giants of the past have sat and studied The Word, physicians have taken God's wishes and have made them possible. As corny as it may sound, I still think that the physician is God's hand.

The alphabet soup of HMOs is frustrating; it's hard to have them put the dollar sign on much of what we do. Certainly, I have made a very good living out of medicine, but I do not think that anyone can ever say that I compromised morality or the patient's interest one single time at any stage of my career. I feel certain that you will act the same way.

On the eve of your graduation, let me remind you again that the opportunity to practice medicine is one of the greatest gifts that you can ever receive. When you started medical school, I told you that you would be privileged to be able to share the most intimate details of peoples' lives. You would see them physically and emotionally naked and do this with moral and legal permission. You will share a person's darkest secret and because you are a physician, he will have confidence that it is really your secret. Because you are a doctor, you can see a man's wife undressed when under other conditions, he would kill you for that action. You will have people put their young children in your hands with complete confidence that you will make them well and certainly bring them no harm. Please do not ever take any of these privileges for granted.

You worked hard in medical school, but there have been people in the past who have gone to any number of sacrifices to be able to gain admittance to a medical school and then to be able to go through with a career. Some of these people have been the grandfathers of our profession who have given us some of the tools that we take for granted.

Whenever I get disillusioned with all of the complications and criticism in medicine, I think back on what it must have been like to sit by a child with pneumonia, not too many years ago, and have nothing to offer. When I see what we have done, not only through research but also through techniques of good quality care, I feel that the future of our profession is great. I feel particularly good about it when I see people like you and your brother coming along to take over.

Most people never have a chance to make any substantial contribution in anyone's life or in any aspect of the world in which they live. You, as a doctor, will have a chance to do this practically every day of your professional career. You will be able to look back on your life and know that you made the world a much better place because you lived here. Medicine will give you that opportunity.

I have watched you grow up with as much pride as a parent can have for a child. I know that you have always felt that and although we tease each other, you know that my love and respect for you goes far beyond that which a father normally has for his son. While I wish you good luck and love you as a father, I now also greet you as a colleague.

Good luck, Doctor!!!

Epilogue

Return to Pettus

After attending the American College of Allergy meeting in 2002, my wife and I drove from San Antonio to Pettus, Texas, and saw the old place again after more than forty years. The three stores were still there: in a half century, no one had found time or inclination to add a fourth. I introduced myself to the general store's current owner who, of course, had not been born when I had my practice there. He was very interested in knowing that there was once a physician's office on the second floor. In fact, he had never ventured upstairs, nor had anyone else done so in many years. I suggested we go up and visit.

What a surprise! It looked as if no one had entered the office since the day we left town. The same travel posters were on the wall, although they were now dusty and faded. The same paper—store wrapping paper—was on the examining table. The exorbitant fees charged in my practice were listed on the front door: three dollars for an office visit, five dollars for a physical, eight dollars for a house call. There was a sign below the price list suggesting that pregnant women come in for at least one examination prior to their due dates. Home deliveries would be made when possible, and family members who intended to conduct a home delivery, probably without medical assistance, were cautioned to come in for at least some discussion on what to do with unexpected complications, where to go, what interim treatments could be given and, almost more important, what not to do.

Time may have come to a standstill in this Pettus second-floor office, but fortunately medical care had not.

Not long ago, back home in Charleston, I was going through some old boxes in my garage and came upon the wooden sign I'd kept from the Pettus office. The sign had been attached to the front of the general store that made up the building's ground floor. It simply said: "Charles H. Banov, MD, Office upstairs."

Just a few days earlier, an attorney friend and I were talking about our careers. He asked me a very profound question: If I had a few words to put on my tombstone describing what I'd like people to remember about my life and any possible contributions, what would they be? His question reminded me of an old story I had heard years ago. Johnny Cash wrote a song about it.

There was a wonderful old physician in Arkansas whose funeral was attended by everyone in the town where he had practiced. Throughout his career, when his patients couldn't pay, he had continued serving them, even when he had to move his office to a rundown second-floor space. On his grave the people of the town hung his shingle: "Doctor Brown. Office Upstairs."

For now, there is life to be lived, tears to be wiped, smiles to be enjoyed and people to be helped. But when the time comes, the greatest compliment I could ever receive from my family, friends, colleagues or patients would include the words of that wooden sign. Just hang it on the tombstone, and that will be enough: Here lies Charles H. Banov, MD, Office upstairs.

About the Author

C harles H. Banov, MD, was born in Charleston, South
Carolina, and has lived there most of his life, though he has
also traveled and taught in more than seventy-five countries. He
emphatically denies that trouble follows him, though he has in
fact been imprisoned by rebels in Venezuela, threatened by drug
lords in Peru and followed by Soviet Union intelligence officers
in Moscow.

A graduate of Emory University and the Medical College
of South Carolina in Charleston, Dr. Banov is a fellow of
many national and international medical societies, including
the American Academy of Allergy, the American College of
Physicians and the American College of Chest Physicians. He
has served as president of the American College of Allergy and
of Interasma, the international organization of world asthma
and chest physicians. The Boy Scouts of America presented him
with a prestigious medical award, though to his chagrin they took
it back, as he was only twelve years old at the time and therefore
ineligible. He has not yet recovered from the disappointment.

Dr. Banov has lectured on the subject of allergies throughout
the world, though a Moscow audience once confused his
comments on cat allergies with off-color remarks about the
sitting American president. A television reporter excitedly
encouraged him to further discuss ragweed allergies while her
own throat was closing up from severe anaphylaxis.

ABOUT THE AUTHOR

With his wife Nancy Leopold Banov, Dr. Banov has raised four children, one of whom, Pamela, has survived with Rett Syndrome, a severe developmental disorder. Nancy founded the South Carolina Society for Autistic Children, and both she and Dr. Banov have testified before the United States Congress on the subject of special-needs children. They remain vigorous advocates for persons with disabilities.